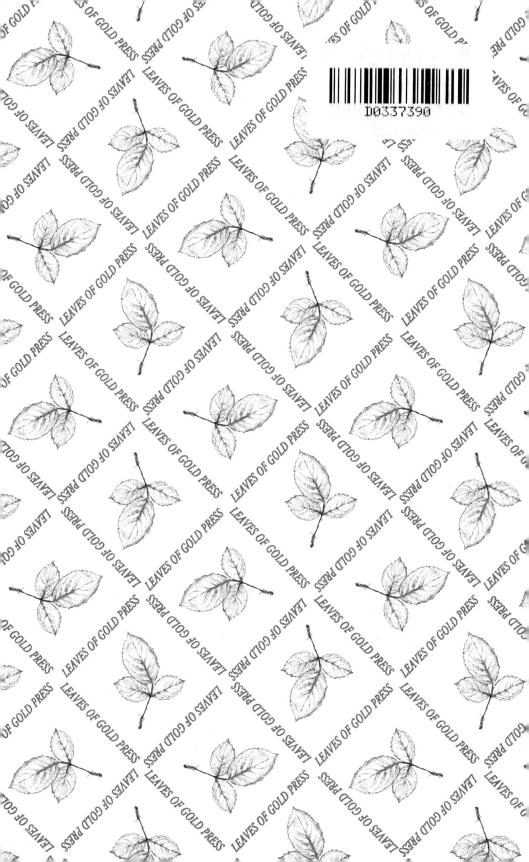

IS
FOOD

MAKING YOU

SICK?

The
Strictly Low Histamine
Diet

James L. Gibb

Revised and updated 2017
Copyright © James L. Gibb 2017
The right of James L. Gibb to be identified as author of this work has been asserted in accordance with the Copyright, Designs and Patents Act, 1988.

National Library of Australia Cataloguing-in-Publication entry

Author: Gibb, James L., author.

Title: Is food making you sick? : the strictly low histamine diet /
James L. Gibb.
Revised 2017 edition.
ISBN: 9781925110500 (paperback)
ISBN: 9781925110999 (hardcover)

Notes: Includes bibliographical references and index.

Subjects: Diet therapy.
Histamine--Toxicology.
Nutritionally induced diseases--Prevention.

Dewey Number: 616.97

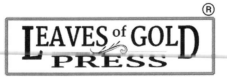

ABN 67 099 575 078

PO Box 9113, Brighton, 3186, Victoria, Australia
www.leavesofgoldpress.com

HOW CAN HISTAMINE INTOLERANCE AFFECT YOU?

SKIN

HIVES

ECZEMA

ITCHING

SKIN RASHES

PSORIASIS

INFLAMMATION

SKIN SENSITIVITY

ACNE (PIMPLES)

EXTREME REACTION
TO INSECT STINGS

STOMACH

NAUSEA

VOMITING

HEARTBURN

ACID REFLUX

STOMACH PAIN

FOOD SENSITIVITIES

BOWEL

DIARRHEA

FLATULENCE

CHRONIC CONSTIPATION

IRRITABLE BOWEL SYNDROME

HEAD & FACE

ASTHMA

HAYFEVER

RUNNY NOSE AND WEEPY EYES,
although there is no clinical sign of allergies

HEADACHES SIMILAR TO MIGRAINE

FLUSHING OF FACE AND/OR CHEST

QUINCKE OEDEMA
(Swellings mostly appearing around eyes and lips,
sometimes in the area of the throat)

OTHER SYMPTOMS

ANXIETY

JOINT PAIN

IRRITABILITY

FUZZY THINKING

SLEEP DISORDERS

FITS OF DIZZINESS

EXTREME TIREDNESS

SEVERE PERIOD PAINS (women)

SUDDEN DROP IN BLOOD PRESSURE

CARDIAC ARRHYTHMIA,
such as a fast beating
or irregular heart beat

Visit the website
www.low-histamine.com

Contents

PART II—Recipes

~ PART I ~

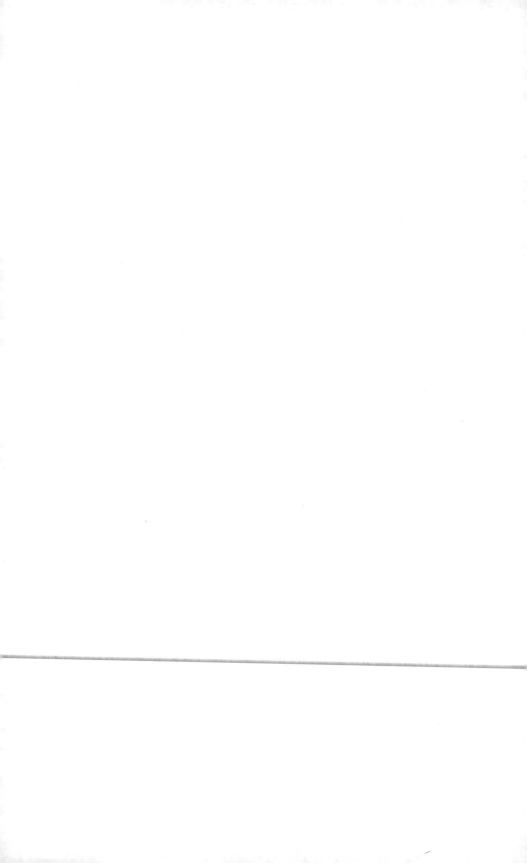

Introduction

People all over the world suffer from histamine intolerance without being aware of it.

We sneeze, suffer from joint pain, inflammation, psoriasis, sleep disorders, irritability, anxiety, bowel disease, diarrhea, flatulence, stomach pain, heartburn and acid reflux, nausea, bloating and other digestive problems, eczema, tissue swelling, urticaria (hives), itching skin, itching scalp, sinusitis, runny nose, puffy eyes, hay fever, asthma, and breathing difficulties, or endure tension headaches, migraines, fuzzy thinking, dizziness, irregular heartbeat, painful periods (women), sudden drops in blood pressure, faintness or flushing, immediately after the consumption of histamine-rich foods, or many hours afterwards. [6]

Like water, histamine is colorless, odorless and tasteless. Unlike water it is invisible and undetectable except by scientific analysis. But it is crucial for life and—like water—under certain circumstances it can kill. [220]

A range of circumstances including our genes, our environment, our diet and stress, cause our bodies' histamine levels to rise. If they rise faster than our bodies can break them down, we experience the excessive inflammation brought on by histamine intolerance, also referred to as histaminosis and HIT.

The good news is, if we can understand what is happening and why, we can treat or prevent this widely unrecognized condition.

BEFORE YOU BEGIN[1]

It can be difficult to diagnose HIT. If you are suffering from any of the symptoms listed in this book, or have been diagnosed with inflammatory bowel disease, it is a good idea to begin by seeking medical advice. Take allergy tests and be screened for any other pathological diseases. If the results are negative and you suspect you are intolerant to histamine, you might consider embarking on a restricted diet to find out whether your symptoms improve.

Because it is practically impossible to avoid all histamine-containing foods, it is recommended that you follow the Strictly Low Histamine Diet while, if necessary, concurrently taking a course of supplements as described in this book.

Be aware that if you are allergic to any of the foods listed in the S.L.H. diet, they will also make your histamine levels rise.

It is important to stringently stick to a low-histamine diet for the initial period. Follow the diet for a minimum of four to six weeks to see if there is any improvement in your health. If you start feeling better, this is an indication that you are indeed histamine intolerant.

Some people will find they need to continue following the SLH diet from a few weeks to several months, depending on their individual symptoms.

Histamine intolerance can be temporary, so after the initial period has elapsed, you may introduce small quantities of higher-histamine foods as a challenge, to test your new toleration threshold. This varies, depending on the individual patient.

James L. Gibb

---

1   Note that the 2017 edition of this book has been updated to reflect the latest research findings. Coconut, which was originally listed as "well-tolerated" by the Swiss Interest Group Histamine Intolerance (SIGHI) and other reputable sources, is no longer recommended for HIT sufferers. It has been added to the "foods to avoid" list. Recipes have been revised accordingly.

1. About Histamine

HISTAMINE IS NECESSARY FOR GOOD HEALTH

Most people are aware of the term 'antihistamine' because it's the active ingredient in medicines that relieve our itches, sneezes, insect stings and allergies in general. But what is histamine?

Histamine occurs naturally in all plants and animals and is actually vital for our good health. On a daily basis, small quantities of histamine are coursing through our blood, keeping us healthy. It is only when the levels rise beyond control that it becomes detrimental.

Our bodies manufacture histamine from the amino acid histidine, which is why it is called a biogenic amine. Histamine is an important excitatory neurotransmitter (a molecule that transmits messages between cells). In addition to its daily duties of defending us against invading toxins, histamine helps to regulate bio-activities as varied as digestion, sleep, blood pressure, sexual function and the operations of the brain.

'Histamine is … involved in local immune responses as well as regulating physiological function in the gut and acting as a neurotransmitter.' [1]

Histamine plays an important role in the body, being involved in at least 23 different physiological functions. [2]

HISTAMINE IS NATURALLY PRODUCED IN OUR BODIES.

When foreign irritants (such as pollen, certain foods, pollution and mosquito saliva) invade our tissues, our immune systems respond. Part of this response involves releasing histamine from storage inside granules that exist in two types of cells. These cells are basophils (a type of white blood cell) and mast cells.

The mast cells occupying connective tissues near the site of the invasion are the ones that produce the histamine, which is why, for example, swelling and redness arise around insect bites and stings. Histamine's job is to trigger this inflammatory response. It 'increases the permeability of the capillaries to white blood cells and some proteins, to allow them to engage pathogens in the infected tissues'. [3]

HISTAMINE RECEPTORS

Histamine performs its various tasks by binding with histamine receptors in our bodies. These receptors, which reside at different locations inside us, are in charge of different physiological functions.

The histamine H1 receptors, for example, control smooth muscle and endothelial cells, thereby influencing our skin and blood vessels. H1 antihistamines such as Benadryl and Claritine inhibit the action of these receptors.

Histamine H2 receptors are situated in the intestines. They are in control of stomach acid secretion, abdominal discomfort, and nausea. They also influence our heart rate. H2 antihistamines such as Ranitidine are prescribed to decrease symptoms of dyspepsia and acid reflux.

In our central nervous system, histamine H3 receptors supervise our nerves, sleep patterns, appetite and behavior. H3 antihistamines have even been suggested as a treatment for obesity. [4]

Our histamine H4 receptors affect the thymus (a specialized organ of the immune system), the small intestine, the spleen, the colon, our bone marrow and our white blood cells. They therefore exert a powerful influence over the function of our immune system and play a role in allergic inflammatory responses. [5]

OTHER HEALTH EFFECTS OF HISTAMINE

Despite the fact that many people endure the negative effects of over-abundant histamine and the resulting inflammation, recent studies indicate that histamine may regulate some forms of cancer growth. [82]

Scientists have discovered that histamine and histamine receptors influence the behavior of cancers of the stomach, pancreas, colon, and liver in various ways. Some cancer cells manufacture a type of histamine called histidine decarboxylase. This inhibits inflammatory cell activity. It is also possible that histamine and mast cells might either encourage or repress cancer in its different phases. Indeed, laboratory tests seem to show that melanoma skin cancer is spurred by histamine and yet curbed by H2 antagonists, histamine-blocking drugs of the type used to treat indigestion, acid reflux and stomach ulcers. [80]

Additionally, researchers are contemplating the use of histamine in preventing the harmful effects of cancer radiation therapy. [81]

It is also possible that histamine guards our bodies by impeding AGE activity [compounds called advanced glycation end products] which contributes to chronic inflammatory diseases such as heart disease, diabetes, brain degeneration and cancer. Studies showed that histamine and H2 receptors repressed the AGE activity that promotes plaque in diabetes. It is postulated that that activating H2 receptors could decrease the risk of atherosclerosis, or hardening of the arteries, which is the leading cause of heart attacks, stroke, and peripheral vascular disease.

2. Histamine Intolerance (HIT)

WHEN CAN HISTAMINE BECOME A PROBLEM?

In most people, histamine molecules have a short life. As soon as they have delivered their chemical message to their target cells, other chemicals produced by the body catabolize them (chemically break them down). They are broken down by two enzymes: histamine-N-methyl transferase (HMT) and diamine oxidase (DAO).

Histamine can be manufactured inside our bodies, or it can enter our systems via histamine-rich foods. Research shows that consuming certain foods can cause a wide range of serious health issues. [7] Some foods, such as tomatoes and spinach, are naturally abundant in histamine.

Part of the problem is that some people don't produce enough HMT and DAO to properly control their histamine levels. DAO occurs abundantly in certain locations – specifically the kidneys, the small bowel and the first section of the large bowel. Its task is to decompose the histamine in our food. If the enzyme is not working properly or if there is not enough of it available, the histamine remains intact and starts to accumulate. This initiates increased inflammation and a wide range of other symptoms, in patterns which vary in each person, and even in each individual flare-up. Consequently, people may suffer the symptoms of excessive histamine or, in some cases, histamine intolerance.

Other causes of overabundant histamine are ingested substances which can block our DAO—such as drugs, certain foods, pollutants or even detergents, which are used as carriers in some medications.

A person who is in good health will only experience a reaction when exceptionally vast quantities of histamine are eaten or released. Although histamine is essential, there is a limit beyond which it is toxic to every animal or human being.

SYMPTOMS OF HISTAMINE INTOLERANCE

Histamine intolerance may be the hidden agent behind malaises such as itchiness, headaches, inability to think clearly, diarrhea, rashes, psoriasis, abdominal pain, gastrointestinal disorders, sneezing, rhinorrhea and congestion of the nose, hives, eczema, asthma, irregular heartbeat, sinusitis, flushing, poor muscle tone, painful periods, flushing and more. These symptoms may manifest themselves soon after exposure to allergens, or many hours later.

'Symptoms can be manifest via the …actions of histamine in multiple organs, such as the gastrointestinum, lung, skin, cardiovascular system, and brain, according to the expression of histamine receptors.' [11]

'These symptoms appear similar to food allergy, sensitivity to sulfites and other "amine" compounds like tyramine.' [9]

In the most serious cases, consuming large amounts of histamine can cause scombroid poisoning, a painful and acutely distressing conditon that can sometimes be fatal.

Excessive levels of histamine can also cause anaphylaxis, the most serious and life-threatening form of response.

THE HISTAMINE CUP

Why does the same food affect people with HIT occasionally, but not every time? Why do their symptoms come and go?

This is because the tide in our histamine 'cup' rises and falls, only causing symptoms after it overflows. When a person's histamine intake exceeds their own tolerance limits, they begin to experience symptoms. Indeed, the fact that histamine intolerance is a dose-related condition is the greatest difference between HIT and allergy.

Imagine that the body is a cup and histamine is water. There is always a small amount of water at the bottom of the cup. This is the essential histamine, made by the body to assist with protection from allergens, the functioning of the brain and the functioning of the digestive system.

If a person with allergies is exposed to allergens (such as insect stings or inhaled pollen, for example), their body releases more histamine. The level of water in the cup rises a little.

The same person may then come into contact with something else to which they are allergic, such as wool, or dust mites. The level rises further.

They may also be eating a high histamine diet, containing foods such as cheese, pickles, tomatoes, shellfish and salami, or beverages such as wine or soft drinks. Each of these foods is contributing to the quantity of liquid in the cup.

If the trend continues and the person adds more and more water to their 'histamine cup', eventually the level will reach the top and overflow. The histamine load has become too great for the body's enzymes to break down the surplus and discharge it via the kidneys. This is the point at which symptoms erupt.

The rim of the cup can be likened to an individual's personal tolerance level. When the cup fills to overflowing, it sets off their symptoms. Thus it is not necessarily a single event, but a set of different events that causes the cup to fill.

LEVELS IN THE BODY'S 'HISTAMINE CUP'

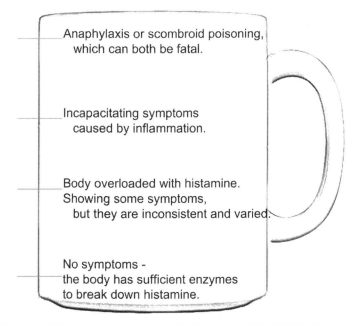

Anaphylaxis or scombroid poisoning, which can both be fatal.

Incapacitating symptoms caused by inflammation.

Body overloaded with histamine. Showing some symptoms, but they are inconsistent and varied.

No symptoms - the body has sufficient enzymes to break down histamine.

EVEN A NORMAL MEAL CAN TRIGGER SYMPTOMS.

'Histamine in food at non-toxic doses has been proposed to be a major cause of food intolerance, causing symptoms like diarrhea, hypotension, headache, pruritus and flushing.

'75 mg of pure liquid oral histamine—a dose found in normal meals—can provoke immediate as well as delayed symptoms in 50% of healthy females without a history of food intolerance.' [192]

VARYING RESPONSE TIMES

Some people suffer an immediate or early reaction to raised histamine levels, while others may experience a delayed reaction that might manifest many hours later. Symptoms of a deferred reaction may last up to 24 hours.

VARYING DEGREES OF SEVERITY

Histamine intolerance symptoms can range from mild to severe. Some people are only slightly affected, and merely notice it now and then. Others are highly sensitive, and even the tiniest deviation from a strict low histamine diet may cause a drastic reaction. The progression from 'susceptible' to 'not susceptible' can be pictured as a continuous line.

'Reactions to histamine described in the literature vary from subjective reports of a wide variety of variable symptoms to full-blown toxicity.' [8]

FOOD ALLERGY OR HISTAMINE INTOLERANCE?

Histamine reactions imitate allergic reactions, making it hard to untangle the two, but a difference does exist. Food allergy is not the same as food intolerance. With a food allergy, the body's immune system responds abnormally to certain foods which may not be intrinsically harmful, and may have no negative effect on other people. The reaction of each individual may vary from slight to serious or even potentially fatal (anaphylaxis). Allergic reactions tend to begin happening sooner than intolerance reactions, which may not develop until some hours after eating. With allergies, even a minuscule portion of the food allergen can result in an allergic reaction.

Food intolerance, on the other hand, occurs when the body has trouble assimilating specific substances in food, or because specific substances have some immediate effect on the body. Food intolerance can produce symptoms similar to those of food allergy, including stomach pain, diarrhea and bloating—nonetheless, the immune system does not participate in food intolerance as it does with the allergic response. Food intolerance is never life-threatening, but it can result in severe symptoms, despite the fact that it is not associated with the immune system. Food intolerance is also different from food allergies in that the response is cumulative, not immediate. Examples include lactose intolerance and intolerance of certain food additives such as monosodium glutamate.

Skin prick allergy tests performed on people who are deficient in DAO and/or who suffer from histamine intolerance are negative, despite the fact that they have allergic-type responses to foods. That is to say, their IgE (immunoglobulin E) levels are not elevated, as they would be if their immune system was overreacting to environmental antigens. [9]

Histamine is involved in both food intolerance and food allergy. With allergic reactions, the body manufactures various chemicals including histamine, which in itself causes many of the allergy symptoms. Thus antihistamines may be used as a medication for some allergic reactions.

Many of us assume we have food allergies, but few people who experience reactions to food actually have a true food allergy.

'DAO insufficiency and histamine intolerance, though not common, could be the reason why some people still have allergy-type reactions to foods in spite of not having food allergy. It is worth the exploration.' [10]

THE DURATION OF HISTAMINE INTOLERANCE

Researchers estimate that around 80% of people with histamine intolerance are middle-aged. This indicates that HIT is a condition that develops over time, rather than something we sustain from birth. Furthermore, it seems that histamine intolerance can be short-lived in some people, which signifies that it can be 'cured'. [10]

3. Why is HIT Largely Unrecognized?

The idea of histamine intolerance is seldom considered by physicians, despite the fact that it is distinctly described in scientific research papers. Histamine intolerance is generally misunderstood or underestimated. People tend to alleviate their symptoms with drugs such as antihistamines, antacids or pain-killers. These medications, while valuable, do not treat the cause of the problems. HIT is largely unrecognized because it is hard to diagnose.

A CONFUSING RESEMBLANCE TO FOOD ALLERGY

Histamine overload symptoms resemble food allergy symptoms, which is why HIT is often misdiagnosed.

SYMPTOMS ARE VARIED AND INCONSISTENT

'... because of the multifaceted nature of the symptoms, the existence of histamine intolerance has been underestimated, and further studies based on double-blind, placebo-controlled provocations are needed.' [11]

However, even randomized, double-blind, placebo-controlled cross-over research studies fail to reproduce single symptoms when oral doses of histamine are given. [6]

THE REACTION IS CUMULATIVE

Histamine intolerance differs from food allergies or sensitivities because the reaction depends on a cumulative dose, and is not immediate. When the 'histamine cup' is full to the brim, even a tiny droplet of water (histamine) will make it overflow, triggering symptoms. However, when the cup is half empty, it takes more water to reach the top. This means that histamine intolerance can be difficult to identify.

INDIVIDUAL TRIGGER LEVELS ARE VARIABLE AND INCONSISTENT

The amount of histamine necessary to trigger symptoms varies for each person. 'In histamine-sensitive patients with reduced DAO activity, symptoms occur even after the ingestion of the small amounts of histamine that are well tolerated by healthy persons.' [11]

TESTING IS DIFFICULT

Histamine intolerance is not a true allergy, and therefore it does not show up on allergy tests.

'Histamine intolerance' describes the body's response to foods with high levels of histamine. 'Allergic reaction' describes what happens when the body itself produces high levels of histamine in response to an allergen (food or something else) it perceives as an invader. That said, sometimes the body's histamine levels are raised due to an allergy.

Allergy testing is easy and lucrative for the medical profession. By contrast, screening for histamine intolerance is fraught with difficulties.

Unlike allergy testing, confirming a serious histamine intolerance isn't easy or profitable for doctors. A 2011 study revealed that 'histamine-intolerant subjects reacted with different organs on different occasions.' [6]

Every histamine intolerant person has a characteristic pattern of symptoms which may not always arise in the same part of the body or at the same severity. The only real test for histamine intolerance necessitates a scrupulous histamine-free diet succeeded by a double-blind food challenge. (See glossary.)

HISTAMINE LEVELS IN FOODS ARE VARIABLE AND INCONSISTENT

The quantity of histamine in foods varies not only over time, but also between various locations within the same food item and between various foods in the same batch.

'When testing histamine levels in different foods, the concentration of histamine can vary considerably between different sampling sites in a single fish, or between individual cans in a single lot.' [12]

4. What Causes Our Histamine Levels to Rise?

Normally, histamine enters our bloodstreams either by being ingested (eaten) or by being released via the body's natural processes.

It can be broken down either by DAO or by histamine antagonists (antihistamine medications).

In general, our histamine levels rise and fall depending on these variables.

Many factors influence the body's histamine levels. Allergens and pollution, food, medications, stress, heat and cold, hormones and nutritional deficiencies all have a considerable effect on our daily histamine fluctuations. But what can cause the levels to rise beyond our tolerance limit?

FOOD

Eating large amounts of histamine rich foods or foods containing histadine can make us absorb enough histamine to experience symptoms similar to an allergic reaction. [87]

High histamine levels in foods can actually cause food poisoning.

'Histamine poisoning is a foodborne chemical intoxication resulting from the ingestion of foods containing excessive amounts of histamine. Although commonly associated with the consumption of [high histamine] scombroid-type fish, other foods such as cheese have also been associated with outbreaks of histamine poisoning. Fermented foods such as wine, dry sausage, sauerkraut, miso, and soy sauce can also contain histamine along with other biogenic amines.' [18]

The symptoms of histamine poisoning are similar to food allergy symptoms, which is why it is frequently misdiagnosed.

Histamine is in so many foods that it cannot be avoided like lactose or gluten. We can, however, ameliorate symptoms by eating low histamine foods.

Freshness Affects Histamine Levels

Histamine develops in food due to microbial enzymes converting the amino acid histidine, which exists in all proteins, to histamine.

When animals are killed—be they meat animals, fish or fowls—bacteria immediately begin to break down the amino acids in the dead tissue. One of the by-products of the 'breaking down' process is histamine. Only by eating or freezing the dead flesh can this process be halted, and the longer the flesh is left uneaten or unfrozen, the more histamine builds up.

Human beings and other animals manufacture DAO in the body. This breaks down the histamine in the meat they eat. However, in dead flesh there is no DAO, so histamine builds up over time. Scavenger animals in the wild—such as vultures, blowflies and hyenas—can tolerate the huge amounts of histamine in rotting carcasses; but human systems are not built to withstand such exorbitant levels.

Histamine cannot be detected by tasting or smelling the meat, because it has no odor or flavor, but the longer meat, fish or poultry remains in storage, unfrozen, the higher rises its levels of biogenic amines. For this reason, histamine is found chiefly in aged, cured, fermented, cultured, and spoiled foods. These histamine-laden foods have turned into potential allergens.

'Foods exposed to microbial contamination also contain histamine in levels determined by the extent and rate of action of the microbes. Histamine levels reach a reactive level long before any signs of spoilage occur in the food. This characteristic has important implications in fin fish, where bacteria in the gut are particularly active in converting histidine to histamine. The longer the fish remains ungutted, the higher the levels of histamine in the flesh.' [17]

Most fresh vegetables have low histamine levels, with the exception of tomatoes, eggplant and other members of the family Solanaceae, and spinach. Meats such as beef and chicken are low in histamine when they are very fresh. Pre-chopped, minced or ground beef, however, is high in histamine, as are pre-sliced, packaged salad vegetables. Very fresh fish is low in histamine, but canned tuna's levels can be exorbitantly high. Anything that has been processed before it reaches your plate is likely to be high in histamines.

The enzyme that transforms histidine into histamine is called HDC. It is able to linger in foods even after the bacteria or yeast that manufactured it have perished, but it be rendered inactive by one to two weeks in the deep freeze. Cooking demolishes it entirely. Unfortunately, once histamine has been produced it cannot be eliminated. Neither cooking, freezing, hot smoking, nor canning gets rid of it. What's more, other indications of spoilage may not accompany excessive histamine levels; consequently those levels may be undiscoverable other than by chemical analysis.

Fermentation Affects Histamine Levels

'Aged protein-containing foods and fermented foods commonly have increased histamine levels. ... All foods subjected to microbial fermentation in the manufacturing process contain histamine. Included in this category are cheeses, fermented soy products, other fermented foods (e.g. sauerkraut), alcoholic beverages, and vinegars.' [17]

Biogenic Amines and Polyamines

Scientists are discovering that histamine and its toxic effects can be influenced by associated compounds in its tribe of biogenic amines including cadaverine, putrescine and tyramine. These can block the catabolism of histamine and contribute to symptoms of intolerance.

In foods, the most prevalent biogenic amines are histamine, tyramine, tryptamine, cadaverine, spermine, putrescine, spermidine, agmatine and 2-phenylethylamine. Dopamine and octopamine have also been discovered in fish, meat and meat products. The breakdown of amino acids in food to form biogenic amines can cause people to suffer allergic-type reactions, with symptoms such as breathing problems, rashes, itching, fever, vomiting, nausea and high blood pressure.

If you noticed a similarity between the term 'putrescine' and the word 'putrid', and between 'cadaverine' and 'cadaver', you are correct. Merriam-Webster defines putrescine as a '...slightly poisonous ptomaine that … occurs widely but in small amounts in living things, and is found especially in putrid (rotting and smelly) flesh.' Cadaverine is formed by the actions of bacteria in dead and decaying bodies. In other words, these clandestine allies of histamine intolerance are found in meat, fish, cheese and deteriorating foodstuffs. The offensive odor of rotting flesh is chiefly due to these two compounds.

'Putrescine … is a foul-smelling organic chemical compound … that is related to cadaverine; both are produced by the breakdown of amino acids in living and dead organisms and both are toxic in large doses.' [20]

Putrescine has the ability to dislodge histamine from its contact with the intestinal muscosa. This in consequence, can boost the levels of free histamine ready to be absorbed into the circulatory system. Grapefruit juice, orange juice and cooked soybeans have been shown to contain high levels of putrescine.

Tyramine-rich foods—including soy sauce, high-protein foods that have been in storage for a long period, aged cheese, meats, fish and red wine—can cause a buildup of tyramine in people with reduced levels of monoamine oxidase (MAO). High levels of tyramine in the body have been associated with migraines.

Aged cheddar cheese is rich in all three polyamines, showing how fermentation and storage can dramatically affect their levels in many foodstuffs.

Other compounds in this group include spermidine and spermine, which are abundant in lentil soup and cooked soybeans.

Incidentally, studies have linked elevated polyamines (putrescine, spermidine, and spermine) in the body with cancers of the colon, breast, lung, prostate and skin. [21]

Numerous spices act to decrease the action of polyamines. On the other hand some substances like curcumin, which is found in turmeric, may also impede the release of DAO. Like histamine, biogenic amines can be generated by bacteria in food but cannot be destroyed by cooking or freezing.

Oxalates and Other Histamine-Releasers

The problem is not merely over-abundant histamine and amines in food. It is also thought that some foods are naturally high in histamine-releasing agents; substances that provoke the body's mast cells into releasing histamine. Oxalates, which occur naturally in plants and animals, may be among these substances. No recognised studies confirmed this, but many patients believe there is a connection.

'Foods that have been reported to release histamine directly from mast cells include uncooked egg whites, shellfish, strawberries, tomatoes, fish, chocolate, pineapple and alcohol.' [17]

Benzoates and Other Food Additives

Benzoates are chemicals used by many industries to arrest spoilage in a vast array of processed foods and personal products such as toothpaste and deodorants. Large quantities of benzoates also exist naturally in particular foods such as prunes, peaches, papaya, pumpkin, soy beans, spinach, strawberries, raspberries, red beans, avocado, berries and nectarines, mixed spice, cinnamon powder, cloves, aniseed, curry, ginger and chilli powder.

'A number of food additives such as azo dyes and preservatives mediate the release of histamine. Some of these chemicals such as benzoates occur naturally in foods, especially fruits, and may have the same effect as the food additive in releasing histamine.' [17]

REDUCED OR INHIBITED ENZYMES DAO AND HNMT

A frequent cause of overabundant histamine and HIT is a deficiency of enzymes diamine oxidase (DAO), an enzyme found in the intestinal mucosa, and histamine-N-methyltransferase (HMT). These are the enzymes that are meant to control histamine levels by chemical decomposition. [83] [11]

'Sensitive persons, with insufficient diamine oxidase activity, suffer from numerous undesirable reactions after intake of histamine containing foods.' [84]

DAO deficiences may be responsible for a misdiagnosis of food allergies. [86]

' ... when activity of either of these enzymes is insufficient, the resulting excess of histamine may cause numerous symptoms resembling an allergic reaction.

'Low levels of DAO and HMT may be genetically inherited from our ancestors, or the enzymes may be blocked by medications, or decreased because of damage to the intestines, or digestive diseases such as celiac and ulcerative colitis. [83]

Histamine intolerance may be caused by abnormally low levels of DAO. DAO is found, among other places, in the membranes of cells lining the small intestine and the upper portion of the colon, therefore people with damaged gastrointestinal systems seem to be at higher risk for histamine intolerance. [85]

BACTERIAL OVERGROWTH

Some medical practitioners hold that one of the main causes of histamine intolerance is the gut's over-production of particular kinds of bacteria which manufacture histamine from food which has not yet been digested. They believe that this causes histamine levels in the digestive tract to increase, overcoming the body's capacity to break down the over-abundant histamine.

ALLERGIES

When we are exposed to allergens, our bodies deliver copious quantities of histamine. The most common allergens include insect stings, animal dander, mold, drugs and chemicals, dust mites, pollen and food. Some immunobiologists now postulate that allergies may have emerged to protect us from environmental toxins. [13]

If your histamine levels are high, it is crucial that you take steps to avoid being exposed to allergens; otherwise your 'histamine cup' will be in danger of overflowing.

Contact allergies, otherwise known as contact dermatitis or skin rashes, may include a vast range of substances such as urushiol (the toxic ingredient in poison ivy), latex, nickel (a metal used in jewelry such as earrings), acrylates (artificial nails), citrus peel, and chemicals added to soaps, sunscreens, shampoos, hair dyes and lotions.

POLLEN AND AIR POLLUTION

Pollution of the air we breathe can cause our histamine levels to rise and increase inflammation in our bodies. This in turn can contribute to cardiovascular disease. Some people are genetically more susceptible to pollution than others.

Research suggests that inhaling 'particulate matter' either for a short time or a long time can exacerbate thrombotic and coagulation tendencies (the formation of blood clots), possibly due to a rise in circulating levels of white cells and platelets and/or histamine and inflammatory cytokines. [14]

Recent studies have revealed that some people suffer inflammation from pollen despite the fact that they have no particular allergy. [15]

WATER POLLUTION

Experiments have demonstrated that the common water contaminants trichloroethylene (TCE) and perchloroethylene (PCE) raised animals' histamine levels by boosting their sensitivity to allergens. These chemical compounds, which industry uses widely in metal degreasing processes, dry cleaning agents, paint removers, adhesives, lubricants and other products, cause harm to the central nervous system and organs such as the liver and kidneys. As a result of their extensive use, TCE and PCE in various concentrations now contaminate our groundwater, drinking water, soil, and air. High exposure to these compounds is toxic, whereas chronic, low-level exposure causes inflammation and damages the human immune system.

We are chiefly exposed to TCE and PCE by breathing contaminated air, consuming contaminated water or dairy products, or using contaminated water for bathing.

'Adverse effects on the immune system resulting from environ-mental pollutants exposure fall within the following immunotoxic effects: allergy hypersensitivity, autoimmunity, and immunosup-pression.' [16]

CONFLICT WITH MEDICATIONS

Even more than food, drugs can hinder our essential hista-mine-catabolizing enzymes, interfering with the physiological process that prevents the body from absorbing too much histamine from food. This escalates the possibility of HIT symptoms. Studies show that non-steroidal anti-inflammatory drugs (NSAIDs), which include ibuprofen, naproxen and aspirin, can trigger an increase in histamine levels and their associated symptoms. [23]

In hospitals, pain-killers and opioid medications are widely used. These drugs release histamine, which causes itching in numerous patients. [24]

Some drugs that cause histamine release or inhibit DAO are listed in the chapter entitled 'Therapies for Histamine Intolerance'.

STRESS

The mast cells in our bodies are activated by stress. [26]] Causes of stress may be environmental, emotional or physical. When mast cells have been activated they release a wide range of inflammatory mediators, which cause or worsen inflamma-tion. These mediator molecules include histamine and cytokines. Cytokines are proteins that can either arouse or impede immune cells. These compounds take a significant part in the evolution of chronic inflammatory diseases such as psoriasis (a skin condition), hair loss, acne, asthma, and inflammatory bowel disease (IBD). Indeed, severe acute stress has been shown to cause histamine levels to rise in mast cells in the colon, consequently disrupting the function of the gastrointestinal system. [27]

HORMONES

High concentrations of histamine have been linked to ascending levels of estrogen. Many women are aware of being more sensitive to histamine and experiencing increased histamine intolerance symptoms during various stages of their monthly ovarian cycle. When women's estrogen levels are high, they are more likely to experience histamine-activated sinus sensitivity. [28] [29]

This may be a two-way process. Histamine apparently encourages a rise in estrogen levels, which in turn aggravates symptoms. During the final phase of the ovarian cycle, diamine oxidase (DAO) levels are elevated. In theory, this should decrease the chance of overabundant histamine throughout that phase.

Estrogens released into our environment by industry may also trigger the release of histamine. Sources include the PVC in plastics, growth hormones administered to food animals, hormones secreted by the animals themselves, and some pesticides.

UNDER-METHYLATION

People with high histamine levels may suffer from a metabolic imbalance caused by under-methylation. These people not only produce too much histamine, they also retain superfluous quantities of it in their blood. This condition is called 'histadelia'. (See glossary.)

Methylation is a vital biochemical mechanism that is necessary for the majority of your body's systems to operate correctly. It takes place billions of times per second, aiding in the daily mending of DNA molecules. It regulates homocysteine, high levels of which are associated with endothelial injury (harm to blood vessels). Methylation also helps to sustain a positive frame of mind, to recover and reprocess molecules that are essential for detoxification, and control inflammation.

'A breakdown in methylation also puts you at higher risk for conditions like osteoporosis, diabetes, cervical dysplasia and cancer, colon cancer, lung cancer, depression, pediatric cognitive dysfunction (mood and other behavioral disorders), dementia, and stroke. And you may be at higher risk for cardiovascular disease.' [30]

5. Disorders Linked to Histamine

ACID REFLUX, HEARTBURN, GASTRIC ACID RELEASE

Gastroesophageal reflux disease, (GERD or GORD) is a painful condition caused by digestive acid rising from the stomach into the esophagus. [75]

Doctors treat this condition with a number of different medicines, among which are antihistamines—specifically H2 blockers, otherwise known as H2-receptor antagonists.

In the stomach, histamine is involved in acid production.

'H2 blockers prevent histamine from landing on H2 receptors. That prevents the stomach from getting the message to make more acid. Therefore, less acid is produced, reducing heartburn. H2 blockers are used to treat both GERD and peptic ulcers.' [76]

Some alternative medicine practitioners believe that many patients diagnosed with GERD may in fact have histamine intolerance instead. [77]

Even the antacids also used to treat GERD work by blocking the H2 receptor and prevent histamine from binding. Both antacids and antihistamines have unwanted side effects, such as reducing folic acid absorption. [78]

Histamine release is halted when the pH of the stomach starts to decrease (i.e. when acidity increases).

ATOPIC ECZEMA

Research shows that patients with atopic eczema (inflammatory dermatitis) generally have high histamine levels and low DAO levels. The symptoms of atopic dermatitis can be reduced with a low histamine diet, even in patients whose food allergy test results are negative. [11]

A study published in 2006 looked at people who had atopic eczema (AE) but who tested negative for food allergies. The rationale for this investigation was the clinical observation that 'in a subgroup of patients with AE, allergy testing proves negative, although these patients report a coherence of food intake and worsening of AE and describe symptoms that are very similar to histamine intolerance (HIT).' [31]

The study concluded that people with atopic eczema who also showed histamine intolerance experienced either total remission or significant improvement in their symptoms after a fortnight on a low histamine diet.

CHEST PAIN

Intravenous injections of histamine have been shown to cause coronary artery spasm in human patients. This temporary, sudden narrowing of one of the arteries that supply blood to the heart impedes or blocks blood flow through the artery and deprives part of the heart of oxygen-laden blood.

'Ginsburg et al. studied 12 patients with nonexertional chest pain who were given intravenous histamine. They demonstrated histamine to be capable of inducing coronary artery spasm. The full potential pathologic significance of histamine-induced coronary artery spasm needs further investigation.' [32]

CHRONIC FATIGUE SYNDROME

It has been suggested that histamine is associated with chronic fatigue syndrome. [33]

COGNITION (MENTAL PROCESSING)

While histamine can stimulate the brain's neurons, it can also suppress those that protect us against any liability to convulsion, drug sensitization, supersensitivity to denervation (where the central nervous system loses control over the muscles), damage caused by a restricted blood supply to tissues, and stress. [70]

DIVERTICULITIS

Sigmoid diverticulitis seems to be more likely in people with a predisposition to allergies. This type of diverticulitis is associated with the inflammation caused by histamine activity. [59]

ERECTION AND SEXUAL FUNCTION

While patients are being treated with courses of of antihistamines such as cimetidine, ranitidine or risperidone, they may experience libido loss and erectile failure. [72]

Furthermore, when histamine is injected into part of the penis, most men whose erectile dysfunction is predominantly owing to psycho-social factors are able to achieve a partial or full erection. [73]

It is thought that H2 antihistamines may cause sexual problems by decreasing the absorption of testosterone. [74]

FIBROMYALGIA

A 2010 study found greatly increased levels of mast cells in the skin of every fibromyalgia patient tested, which clearly suggested a link. [34]

HEMORRHOIDS

Hemorrhoids, or piles, are dilated blood vessels in the rectum or anus. When these vascular structures become swollen and inflamed, they cause pain and discomfort. Their occurrence is linked with mast cells and histamine. [35]

HYPOTHERMIA

Hypothermia is a condition in which the body's core temperature drops below 35.0 °C, which is defined as the required temperature for normal metabolism and body functions. Histamine plays a role in regulating body temperature, which in turn influences various body functions. [56] [57]

One study showed that a diet deficient in vitamin B1 caused hypothermia and an increase in histamine levels. This was reversed when vitamin B1 was added back to the diet. [58]

INFLAMMATION

Many inflammatory diseases are connected with histamine functions. Histamine and its receptors are forever struggling to achieve equilibrium between avoiding too much inflammation on the one hand, and enabling stability and the restoration of health on the other.

For example in periodontitis, a set of inflammatory diseases affecting the gums, there is a high level of histamine in the diseased tissue. The drug cimetidine, an H2 antagonist, is applied topically to greatly relieve symptoms. [36]

Cryotherapy relieves pain in patients with rheumatoid arthritis, which is an inflammatory disease. Studies show that cryotherapy reduces histamine levels for lengthy periods. It is thought that particular histamine receptors in joint tissues are linked to chronic diseases such as arthritis. [37]

INFLAMMATORY BOWEL DISEASE

DAO helps with the integrity of the gut lining, protecting us from leaky gut and the functional digestive issues that can precipitate from it. Patients with these chronic inflammatory bowel diseases have reduced levels of DAO enzymes in their gut, which suggests histamine intolerance. [9]

Studies also show that between the gut of healthy people and the gut of patients with ulcerative colitis and Crohn's disease, there are significant differences in the distribution and amount of histamine released. [38]

Inflammatory mediators such as histamine, released from intestinal mast cells, may trigger the inflammatory process of inflammatory bowel diseases. [65]

MEMORY

Studies suggest that histamine controls the systems by which memories and learning are forgotten. [71]

MÉNIÈRE'S DISEASE

Ménières Disease involves an overabundance of fluid in the inner ear. The superfluous fluid upsets the ear's balance and hearing mechanisms. Typical symptoms of Ménière's disease include chronic vertigo (dizziness), nausea and/or vomiting, possibly diarrhea, fluctuating hearing loss, tinnitus (a ringing sound in the ears), and a feeling of pressure or fullness in the ear. [60]

The condition is associated with histamine levels. Histamine triggers inflammation, which in turn produces fluid. When the fluid is confined in the small interior of the inner ear, problems arise. The fluid, unable to escape, compresses nerves and soft tissue, affecting both balance and hearing. [62]

One of the treatments for the disease is a drug called beta-histidine, whose chemical structure closely resembles that of phenethylamine and histamine. Betahistidine's action is to repress histamine H3 receptors while stimulating H1 receptors.

'... betahistine is effective in the treatment of Ménière's disease and related conditions.' [61]

MIGRAINES

Research indicates a strong link between migraines and allergies. The blood plasma of migraine patients typically has raised levels of histamine.

'Headache can be induced dose-dependently by histamine in healthy persons as well as in patients with migraine. ... Many migraine patients have histamine intolerance evidenced by reduced DAO activity, triggering of headache by food rich in histamine (e.g. long-ripened cheese or wine), and the alleviation of headache (ie, disappearance of symptoms) under a histamine-free diet and therapy with antihistamines.' [11]

The antihistamine medications which are aimed at histamine H1 and H2 receptors have been ineffective at easing the symptoms of migraine, so more recent studies are focusing on histamine H3 or H4 receptors with hope for improved outcomes.

MOTIVATION AND ADDICTION

High levels of histamine in the brain may affect addiction and alcohol dependence. Brain histamine plays a pivotal role in motivation. 'Motivation' includes activities such as the investigation of new surroundings, procreation, nurturing of offspring, and reactions to dangerous situations. Evidence suggests that impairment of the histamine system may be at the root of some types of apathy and eating disorders.

It is also thought that there may be a strong association between brain histamine and drug addiction. [39]

MULTIPLE SCLEROSIS

Research has demonstrated that histamine receptors play a part in multiple sclerosis. Some receptors stimulate the disease while others repress it. [40]

OBESITY, HEART DISEASE AND DIABETES

Research indicates that mast cells supply various secretions that add to the inflammatory processes associated with coronary artery disease, diabetes and obesity. [79]

OSTEOPOROSIS

For the entire duration of our lives, our bodies are continuously remodeling our skeletons; exchanging old bone for new. Bone remodeling is sometimes called 'bone turnover'. Normally the new bone is equivalent in mass to the old, so there is no loss of overall mass. Throughout our childhood and adolescence however, bone formation exceeds bone resorption, resulting in a net increase in bone mass. The opposite occurs as a consequence of diseases such as osteoporosis, leading to a loss of bone mass. [45]

Bone turnover and bone density appear to be affected by mast cells and the compounds they produce, especially histamine. [46]

Female hormones such as estrogen also play a part. In women with low estrogen levels who do not eat enough calcium-rich food, mast cells become activated. The activated mast cells lead to the body reabsorbing its own bones, drawing calcium from them to ensure that there is sufficient calcium in the bloodstream to keep our bodies functioning properly. When calcium is removed from our bones, the result is osteoporosis.

' Estrogen deficiency associated with calcium deficiency can lead to bone resorption through the activation of mast cells.' [47]

Researchers have suggested that inhibiting mast cells and/or their products—such as histamine—might one day be used as a treatment for osteoporosis. [48]

PARKINSON'S DISEASE, ALZHEIMER'S DISEASE AND BRAIN DEGENERATION

Inflammation triggered by excessive histamine can harm neurons in the brain. Evidence reveals that patients with Parkinson's disease have an unusually diminished capacity to dismantle histamine in the brain, and a build-up of histamine methyltransferase. [50]

The histaminergic system has a role in the treatment of brain disorders, and researchers hope that histamine could be an effective therapeutic factor in the treatment of Alzheimer's disease. [49]

PSORIASIS

Scientific tests conducted on human beings showed that treatment of psoriasis patients with antihistamines significantly improved their symptoms. The researchers concluded that histamine may be involved in the pathophysiology of psoriasis. [221]

RISK OF DISEASE

Too much histamine increases the permeability of the blood-brain barrier, which can make us susceptible to diseases such as bacterial infections. Rifts in the blood-brain barrier are involved in the evolution of epilepsy, Alzheimer's Disease, meningitis, and multiple sclerosis. [63] [64]

SCHIZOPHRENIA

The brain and spine fluid of patients with schizophrenia contain high levels of chemical compounds produced by the breakdown of histamine. Simultaneously, their H1 receptors are less effective. Histamine's use appears to be out of kilter in schizophrenics; thus doctors sometimes prescribe antipsychotic medications with the effect of antihistamines. [69]

SCOMBROTOXIC POISONING

Numerous cases of what is thought to be food poisoning are in fact the result of the consumption of high-histamine foods, rather than foods contaminated only with bacterial pathogens. Scombroid food poisoning, for example, is caused by ingesting fish that is no longer fresh. Decaying fish contains harmful levels of histamine.

Scombrotoxic poisoning is also termed histamine poisoning, because histamine is its chief constituent. 'Other biogenic amines in spoiled fish, such as putrescine and cadaverine, may act as potentiators for histamine toxicity.' [43]

Scombrotoxin's name derives from the fact that it is usually caused by consumption of scombroid fish—species belonging to the Scombridae and Scomberesocidae families, especially tuna, skipjack, bonito and mackerel.

When consumed in adequate amounts, scombrotoxin causes symptoms to evolve swiftly—usually from 10 minutes to 2 hours after the meal. The array of symptoms is quite extensive, and may include burning or tingling of the mouth, or a peppery taste; red skin rashes, hives, itching and localized inflammation, headaches, a sudden drop in blood pressure leading to faintness, headaches and flushing (becoming red in the face). Some patients may develop nausea, vomiting and diarrhea. Hospitalization may be necessary for elderly or sick people. In general, however, the symptoms dissipate within 24 hours.

Scombrotixin, however, is not limited to scombroid fish. Non-scombroid fish, such as sardines, herring, pilchards, marlin and mahi-mahi have been associated with outbreaks of poisoning. [41] Scombrotoxin can also occur in salmon. [42]

The toxin can occur in fish that is fresh, frozen, canned or cured.

Scombrotoxic poisoning is often misdiagnosed because of the resemblance of its symptoms to an IgE-mediated allergic response. Nonetheless, it is believed that histamine poisoning is one of the most prevalent types of fish-related toxicity.

Proper handling and prompt refrigerated storage can discourage histamine formation in fish. [43] [44]

SLEEP DISORDERS

The fact that first-generation H1-targeting antihistamines (see glossary) had the side effect of making patients drowsy proved that histamine plays a role in keeping people awake and vigilant.

If the histamine releasing neurons in our brains were to be destroyed, we would find it impossible to remain alert.

Furthermore, studies show that antihistamines targeting the H3 receptors increase wakefulness. If any of these receptors become damaged or destroyed for any reason, histamine regulation is disrupted, and permanent sleep disorders may result.

'It has been shown that histaminergic cells have the most wakefulness-related firing pattern of any neuronal type thus far recorded. They fire rapidly during waking, fire more slowly during periods of relaxation/tiredness and completely stop firing during REM and NREM (non-REM) sleep.' [51]

H3 receptor antihistamines may prove to be an efficacious treatment for unwanted sleepiness.' [53]

VERTIGO, MOTION SICKNESS AND NAUSEA

Histamine is associated with afflictions such as dizziness, vertigo, nausea, motion sickness and other problems relating to the sense of balance. In hospitals, antihistamines are used to treat post-operative nausea and vomiting. [55]

'Sedating antihistamine medications such as promethazine work quite well for motion sickness, although they can cause significant drowsiness.' [54]

6. Therapies
for Histamine Intolerance

'Many factors affect the body's histamine levels, and there are ways we can help reduce the load. Our exposure to allergens, diet, drug use, temperature, hormones, and nutritional deficiencies dramatically impact our histamine levels throughout the day. Imagine your histamine as a "bucket" that fills up and only reveals symptoms after overflowing.' [11]

TEMPORARY IMMEDIATE RELIEF

Cortisone cream provides a quick fix for skin reactions such as rashes, itching, lumps, eczema and swelling. Applied topically it relieves itching and may aid in the prevention of infection. It should not, however, be used long-term.

Pills and nasal sprays containing corticosteroids may be used to provide immediate relief for some allergy symptoms. Again, they are not intended for prolonged use, as their side effects are potentially injurious or even fatal.

Oral and topical antihistamines can give swift relief from insect stings, allergic reactions etc. They, too, should not be used over a long period, because they interfere with many physiological processes.

Instead of relying on medications to allay our unpleasant signs of histamine intolerance, we can reduce our histamine load in a number of ways, so that our histamine cup never again overflows and we can enjoy life symptom-free.

LOW HISTAMINE NUTRITION

Choose low histamine or antihistamine foods rich in vitamins and minerals.

Consuming a diet rich in natural antihistamines can help prevent histamine intolerance symptoms from occurring.

Eating foods rich in vitamins (especially B-group, E and C), minerals, omega-3 and flavonoids such as quercetin can reduce our histamine load.

If our bodies are deficient in copper, vitamin C and B vitamins such as B6, B12 and folate, they may be unable to decompose histamine sufficiently to defeat symptoms of intolerance.

B vitamins

These are found in whole, unprocessed foods, such as whole grains and eggs (avoid egg whites: eat only the yolks). Vitamin B rich foods also include potatoes and sunflower seeds, but beware; sunflower seeds are high in histamine, while some foods, including potato, are also rich in oxalate, which can release histamine in some people. Folate-rich foods such as whole grains are important for those who suffer from under-methylation.

C vitamins

C vitamins (also called 'ascorbic acid') are found in most fresh vegetables and fruits. Vitamin C is especially beneficial to people with HIT because studies have shown that it may increase the activity of the DAO enzyme. [88]

Be careful—despite the fact that while citrus fruits and spinach are high in vitamin C, they also release histamine in the body and may exacerbate symptoms.

Foods containing abundant in Vitamin C should be consumed when fresh, because the vitamin loses its potency after exposure to air, or after processing, cooking, or long-term storage. Foods rich in vitamin C include cauliflower, parsley, broccoli, mustard greens, watercress, cabbage, turnips, Brussels sprouts, asparagus, cantaloupe, mango, green onions, green peas, radishes, yellow summer squash, sweet potatoes, new potatoes (unless you are sensitive to oxalates), lettuce, honeydew melon, rutabaga, and kohlrabi.

Copper

Our bodies need copper to create the DAO enzyme. Foods high in copper include many that are, unfortunately, also high in histamine, such as sundried tomatoes, crustaceans, cocoa powder, cashews, shellfish, herbal tea, sesame seeds, beans, and lentils. Fortunately copper is also found in low histamine foods such as fresh basil, barley, chives and leeks.

Zinc, calcium and magnesium

Trace minerals, especially zinc, calcium and magnesium, also help combat HIT. Foods rich in zinc include egg yolks and oats. Calcium is abundant in many foods, such as dark leafy greens, okra, broccoli and green beans. Remember that our bodies cannot absorb it without the presence of vitamin D, whose natural source is sunshine. Dark leafy greens provide plentiful magnesium, as do whole grains such as brown rice.

Flavonoids, especially quercetin

Flavonoids, such as quercetin, are a collection of plant pigments that produce colors found in many fruits, vegetables, leaves, grains and flowers. Quercetin is a powerful, natural antihistamine that helps stabilize mast cells to prevent both the manufacture and release of histamine, as well as other allergic and inflammatory compounds. Good sources of quercetin are onions, garlic, apples, parsley, broccoli and lettuce.

Apples, especially apple pectin

Apples (Malus domestica) are a good source of antioxidants, flavonoids such as quercetin, vitamin C and dietary fiber. They are also very low in histamine, saturated fat, cholesterol and sodium. Apples are a versatile fruit which can be eaten raw, or used in baked goods, salads, sauces and desserts.

Research has shown that apple pectin can obstruct the absorption of food allergens. [116]

Fruit pectin has been used to treat high cholesterol, diabetes and gastroesophageal reflux disease (GERD). It binds substances in the intestine, and has also been used to help prevent colon cancer.

Instructions on how to extract pectin from apples, to use in cooking can be found here: ["Make Your Own Apple Pectin" on page 230.]

Rice bran, especially black rice bran

Bran is the outer husk of a cereal grain. Studies suggest that rice bran, especially the bran from black rice, suppresses the release of histamine. Rice bran is low in cholesterol and sodium, a good source of potassium, zinc and copper, and very rich in dietary fiber, B-vitamins, iron, magnesium, phosphorus and manganese.

Anti-allergenic

Certain cultivars of black rice bran have the potential to protect against allergic diseases such as hay fever and asthma and allergic dermatitis symptoms, such as swelling. [117]

In fact, in November 2011 the Korea Food Research Institute filed a patent for 'novel use of rice, rice bran or rice hull extract as a histamine receptor antagonist', stating that ' ... rice, rice bran or rice hull extract can be used as a natural antihistamine, 'to prevent or treat allergic rhinitis, inflammatory bowel disease, asthma, bronchitis, nausea, gastric and duodenal ulcer, gastro-esophageal reflux disease, sleep disorder, anxiety and depression. ... Derived from the natural product rice, rice bran or rice hull, it has no side effect such as cognitive impairment, resistance or dependency even after long-term use.' [118]

Anti-inflammatory

Studies have found that black rice bran inhibits the release of histamine, thereby averting inflammation. [120] Inflammation is often the cause behind a number of body ailments, including allergies, asthma, cardiovascular diseases, cancer and even aging. In a study published in the American Chemical's Journal of Agricultural and Food Chemistry, researchers found that mice fed with a diet supplemented with 10 percent black rice bran significantly reduced inflammation of the ear skin compared to mice fed on standard diet or ones supplemented with 10 percent brown rice bran. [119]

Indeed, all pigmented (colored) rice brans have beneficial effects. on human health. Their bioactivities include antioxidant and free radical scavenging, antitumor, antiatherosclerosis, hypoglycemic, and antiallergic activities. Anthocyanins are considered to be major functional components of pigmented rice. [132] Pigmented rices include black, brown, purple and red.

Cooked broccoli

Broccoli contains calcium, vitamin C, B vitamins and folate, which are all beneficial for sufferers of HIT. It is also low in saturated fat and cholesterol, while being a good source of protein, iron, phosphorus, dietary fiber, magnesium, vitamin A, vitamin E (alpha tocopherol), vitamin K, potassium and manganese. Raw broccoli can be fairly high in oxalates, so it is best to eat it steamed.

HISTAMINE AVOIDANCE

Steer clear of foods rich in histamine, histamine liberators, DAO blockers, biogenic amines and vitamin depleters.

Avoid fermented foods

Fermented foods are high in histamine. These include aged or smoked meats, vinegar (including pickles, prepared mustard and ketchup), sauerkraut, wine, fermented soy products (including tofu and soy sauce), and aged cheese.

Avoid foods exposed to high levels of bacteria

These include fish and shellfish (which may easily be contaminated by their own gut bacteria after death), and leftover meats.

Bacteria can also manufacture histamine. 'Bacterial HDC [histidine decarboxylase] can also convert histidine into histamine, and bacterial infection of food can result in elevated levels of histamine, which can in turn cause food poisoning.' [25]

Avoid foods naturally high in histamine

Foods naturally high in histamine include wheat-based products (wheat germ has high levels of histamine), prepackaged meals, beans, pulses, nuts, tea (herbal or standard) and soy milk. See the chapter entitled 'The Food List' for more details.

Avoid foods rich in histamine liberators

Foods that may stimulate the release of histamine include citrus fruits, nuts, pumpkin, strawberries, chocolate, cocoa, eggplant, tomato, spinach, and spices such as cloves, cinnamon and chili powder.

Foods high in animal fat should be avoided also. Research suggests that fat absorption may drastically boost the release of histamine and encourage chronic inflammation. [89] [90]

Avoid foods high in histadine

Foods containing relatively large amounts of histadine may also cause problems, because histadine is converted to histamine. Such foods include cottage cheese, game meat (venison, buffalo, elk, moose, caribou etc.), pork (loin, chops or other cuts, ham, bacon etc.), soy protein, chicken, turkey, veal, beef, pastrami, lamb, cheese, raw egg whites, bananas, sesame seeds, sunflower seeds, mustard seed, seaweed, cottonseed flour, codfish, soy protein and yeast.

The bacteria in the gut of fin fish are especially active in converting histidine to histamine. The longer the fish remains ungutted, the higher soar the levels of histamine in the flesh. The term 'fin fish' is used to describe seafood with fins. Fin fish are also referred to as 'true fish'. Examples of aquatic animals that are not fin fish are shellfish and crayfish. Fin fish include such creatures as perch, grouper, pike, cod, sunfish and tuna.

Avoid foods that interfere with the body's ability to break down histamine.

These foods include alcohol and animal fats.

Avoid preserved foods, especially those containing benzoates.

Benzoates are chemicals that are industrially used to preserve food. They can trigger histamine release. Preservatives artificial flavorings and colorants can trigger mast cell histamine release. [91]

Avoid excessive sugar and saturated fat

Sugar and saturated fat have been shown to deplete the body's reserves of vitamins.

For more information about how to reduce your food-related histamine load, see our chapter entitled The Strictly Low-Histamine Diet [page 81].

A NATURAL SOURCE OF DAO

Pea sprouts to boost your DAO

When our diamine oxidase enzyme levels are low we can suffer from histamine intolerance. A number of legumes contain especially high levels of DAO. Eating these legumes as sprouts can provide us with a natural diamine oxidase boost.

The new seedlings of all legumes can provide us with DAO, but green pea sprouts are the best sources. Lentils and chickpeas are also good.

DAO is high in legume seedlings because the diamine oxidase helps the plant to build its structural components, such as its stem, when the baby plant is forming. Diamine oxidase begins to be produced about three days into the development of the seedlings. It increases to its maximum at about 10 days, after which it decreases because the plant no longer requires it.

Highest possible DAO concentrations

When seeking DAO from natural sources we need to obtain the highest concentrations possible, because the process of digestion itself can destroy the DAO before it works its magic on our histamine levels.

Studies have shown that up to 4% of the total protein content of the seedlings can be diamine oxidase. Histamine intolerance specialist Dr Janice Joneja explains that since diamine oxidase is a protein, the body will try to digest it, thereby breaking it down. One cannot predict how much DAO will be absorbed into the body and how much will remain active to help break down histamine.

Dark-grown sprouts

To increase the levels of DAO in your home-sprouted legumes, grow them in darkness. Sprouts that are grown in the dark have a higher level of diamine oxidase. Diamine oxidase is a protective enzyme for both humans and plants. Thus, when plants experience stress, they produce more of it.

When seeds grow in the dark they have to struggle. This struggle produces a much higher level of diamine oxidase. Dark-sprouted pea shoots will appear lank and pale ('etiolated'. They may not look as vibrant and healthy as green sprouts, but their content of diamine oxidase will be approximately five times higher than the content of bright green seedlings grown in sunlight. They are therefore better for people with histamine intolerance.

About store-bought pea sprouts

It is possible to buy pea sprouts that have been commercially grown and bagged. Eating them may be somewhat beneficial to your health, but they have the following disadvantages:

- Their DAO levels vary greatly
- They may have languished on the shelf for a while, and not be super-fresh. Thus their histamine levels may be high.
- They are generally grown in sunlight or artificial sunlight – that's why they are green. Therefore their DAO levels are much lower.

About store-bought pea sprout powder

Store-bought pea sprout powder can also be used. It is difficult, however, to estimate exactly how much DAO it contains, which means we cannot know what dosage to take on a daily basis for optimum benefit. Dr Joneja recommends mixing a cupful a day with water and taking that, to see if you get any benefit.

Benefits of home-grown pea sprouts

Growing pea sprouts at home has numerous benefits.

- Speed – your crop can be ready for harvest in less than ten days.
- Convenience – they can be grown indoors, and need no soil.
- Economy – you can sprout dried 'soup peas' from the supermarket.
- Higher DAO – grow them in the dark and their enzyme levels will be far higher.
- Flexibility – grow them anytime.
- Compactness – you can grow them in small spaces.
- Flavor – sprouts can be consumed raw in juices.
- Nutrition – in addition to DAO, pea sprouts are packed with vitamins A and C and folic acid.

How to grow pea sprouts/seedlings

Obtain peas that are intended for eating, not for planting. Pea seeds that are sold for planting in gardens may have been dusted with chemicals to inhibit mold or to kill insects. Choose fresh green peas from your greengrocer or dried peas from the grocery section of your supermarket. Do not select dried peas that are salted, frozen, split or processed in any way. Try to find organic peas. Freeze dried peas are fine. (Shop online for them here.)

- To avoid bacterial contamination, do not grow seedlings in soil.
- Do not sterilize the pea seeds. If you heat them, you will deactivate the diamine oxidase enzyme.
- Rinse the peas in clean, cool water.
- Place the peas in a bowl, and cover them with more clean water.

- Allow them to soak for 12-24 hours.
- Place the seeds in a clean seed-sprouting bag or other sprouting equipment (see below) and leave the bag in the dark (such as a drawer or cupboard, or wrapped in a thick towel), for 7-10 days; no later. Do not leave them in the refrigerator – they need to be at room temperature, at least.
- Two or three times a day, rinse them with clean water to hydrate them. Always tip out all of the water to drain the peas thoroughly. Do not forget to rinse them or they may become moldy. One trick for remembering is to rinse them whenever you clean your teeth.
- Continue the process for 8-10 days. Pale shoots will emerge from the peas and start to grow.
- Harvest the sprouts.
- Juice them raw and consume them straight away. Do not heat them – heating destroys DAO.
- Mature sprouts have sets of two leaves. Only mature sprouts should be juiced. Immature sprouts contain an amino acid that can aggravate some health issues.
- Rinse sprouts before for juicing. If you wish, you can wrap them in a lettuce leaf to help the juicing process and make sure the nutrients are extracted.
- Store leftover sprouts in the refrigerator in a sealed bowl containing a paper towel to absorb excess moisture. Use the sprouts within a week.

Note: Sprouts that start to look rather brown in color should be discarded because they are past their use-by date. Over-aged sprouts may also release a yellowish liquid in their container.

Pea-sprouting equipment

- Bags: Seed-sprouting bags are drawstring bags made from a closely-woven, natural fabric (not plastic) such as cotton or hemp. You can make your own or buy them commercially. Seed-sprouting bags are made by stitching together two rectangles of cotton or hemp, with a drawstring opening.
- Jars: The cheapest seed-sprouting equipment is a clean glass jar. Cover the mouth of the jar with clean stockings or pantyhose, held in place by an elastic band. The pantyhose acts as a strainer when rinsing the peas with water.
- Commercial: You can also purchase commercial seed-sprouting equipment. In the electrically-powered versions, the water is automatically filtered through.
- Make sure you position all your sprouting equipment in a pitch dark place while your seeds are growing.

How to use pea sprouts/seedlings

Use your pea sprouts in smoothies, rather than eating them in their unprocessed form. Diamine oxidase enzymes exist to help the plant build the wall of its cells, so they are attached to those cell walls.

Your normal chewing and digestion will not readily break those bonds. By whizzing the sprouts in a blender you will make the DAO more readily available for your body to absorb. Do not put the juice through a strainer – it's vital to consume the whole plant, cell walls, fiber and all. See our recipes here.

One cup every day is the recommended dose.

OTHER THERAPIES FOR HIT

Avoid excessive heat and UVB rays

In some people, exposure to sunshine and heat can exacerbate dermatitis and skin rashes. Research indicates that the sun's shortwave ultraviolet B (UVB) rays causes cells to release histamine in test-tube experiments, despite the cells having been shielded with ascorbic acid (vitamin C). [92] [93]

Exercise sensibly

Fairly vigorous exercise has been known to set off episodes of anaphylaxis, especially in warm surroundings. Usually these severe responses are linked to food allergens that were eaten before the exercise was undertaken. A 2011 study showed that dynamic exercises (such as running, vigorous dancing or jogging) releases the amino acid L-carnosine, which is subsequently converted to histamine. It might be possible to avert symptoms of histamine intolerance arising during physical activity, by rigorously shunning allergens. [94]

Avoid drugs that inhibit DAO or liberate histamine.

In consultation with your medical practitioner, choose compatible alternatives to DAO inhibiting drugs. DAO inhibiting drugs include—but are not limited to—

- MGBG (a drug used to treat cancer)
- MAO inhibitors (drugs used to treat depression)
- acetylcysteine (a cough medicine: eg. Mucomyst, NAC, Acetadote)
- ambroxole (an expectorant; including Mucosolvan, Mucobrox, Mucol, Lasolvan, Mucoangin, Surbronc, Ambolar, Lysopain)
- aminophylline (a bronchodilator: eg. Phyllocontin, Truphylline)
- amitriptyline (antidepressants such as Elavil, Endep, Vanatrip)
- chloroquine (an anti-malarial)
- clavulinic acid (a combination antibiotic)
- isoniazid (a tuberculosis treatment)
- metamizole (a pain reliever and fever reducer)
- metoclopramide (nausea and vomiting medicines)
- propafenone (used to prevent irregular heartbeat)
- verapamil (used to treat high blood pressure and chest pain)

Reduce stress

While stress doesn't actually cause symptoms, it can indirectly trigger them by activating mast cells and increasing the histamine in your bloodstream. When we experience stress, our bodies release a hormone called cortisol. Studies indicate that this hormone seems to boost histamine levels in the stomach and intestines. Likewise a reduction in stress can decrease cortisol, thus diminishing the activation of mast cells and lowering histamine release.

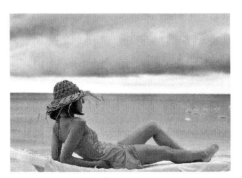

Reduce stress

Sugar and a Low Histamine Diet

"Sugar is the new fat!"

This is the latest slogan popular in the wonderful and sometimes weird (not to mention confusing) world of food fads and fashions.

Fat used to be "bad" and then it became "good". Carbohydrates used to be "good" until they did a 180 degree turn and became viewed as "bad". Hardly anybody used to even know what gluten was until it, too, joined the ranks of "foods to be shunned". Wine keeps switching sides, so that it's sometimes hard to know what to believe.

Not only can food fashions be confusing, they can also be dangerous. Google definitions describes orthorexia as "an obsession with eating foods that one considers healthy," and "a medical condition in which the sufferer system-atically avoids specific foods that they believe to be harmful."

The danger with following too many food-exclusion diets simultaneously, is that people can become orthorexic.

The book is about Histamine Intolerance. It is not about a sugar free diet. It is not about a low-carb, gluten-free, low-FODMAP, lactose-free, vegan, veg-etarian, fruitarian, specific carbohydrate, ketogenic, diabetic, detox, low-fat or any other kind of diet.

It is virtually impossible to cater for the entire range of popular diets, all in one book whose purpose is to focus on histamine intolerance. We have done our best, however! Many of our recipes are gluten-free, dairy-free vegetarian or vegan.

Furthermore, the fact is that sugar is not a food that is high in histamine, or that provokes a histamine reaction in the body, or that blocks the breakdown of histamine.

Having said that, it is important to note that Dr Alison Vickery states that histamine tolerance can be improved through the stabilization of blood sugar levels. She writes, "… unstable blood sugar can increase histamine levels, and histamine levels can progress the development of diabetes or insulin resistance."

So, while sugar as a food in itself is not directly a problem for people with histamine intolerance, eating too much of it can cause a "spike" in your blood sugar levels. A spike is generally followed by a sharp drop in blood sugar levels as the body releases insulin to cope with your sugar intake. These zig-zagging spikes and sharp drops are what is meant by "unstable blood sugar".

To stabilize your blood sugar levels:

- Avoid eating large quantities of sugar and foods containing refined carbohydrates (such as sodas, candy, cakes etc.)
- Choose foods that are low on the glycemic index.
- Avoid artificial sweeteners altogether.
- If you want extra low-calorie sweetness, choose stevia.

Alternatives to Table Sugar

People who prefer to eat less sugar can easily adapt the Strictly Low Histamine Diet to their needs. Here are some suggestions:

- Choose, from this book, recipes that contain no sugar.
- For recipes containing sugar, substitute rice malt syrup. Anti-sugar advocates say that the main problem with sugar is its fructose content. Rice malt syrup (also known as brown rice syrup) is fructose-free.
- Alternatively, substitute stevia for sugar. Stevia is a natural sweetener derived from the "sweet-leaf" plant, and it does not cause a spike in blood sugars when consumed.

SUPPLEMENTS: VITAMINS, MINERALS AND OILS

Medications, or antihistamine and immune-cell stabilizing nutrients such as vitamins and herbs may help ameliorate HIT symptoms; however, drugs and supplements are no substitute for long term, strict compliance with a balanced, low-histamine diet of fresh food. The mainstay of HIT therapy is a sustained and consistent avoidance of foods that trigger symptoms.

Supplements may be used if diet alone is not sufficient for freedom from symptoms of histamine intolerance, or if the temporary low-histamine diet cannot be maintained.

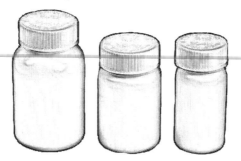

Vitamin C (ascorbic acid)

'Vitamin C is a natural antihistamine. It both blocks histamine release and increases the breakdown of histamine. A 1992 study showed that adults who took 2 grams of vitamin C daily lowered their blood histamine levels by 38 percent in only seven days. [97]

Evidence also shows that low concentrations of serum (blood plasma) vitamin C is correlated with increased serum histamine levels. [98] [99]

Vitamin C is also a powerful antioxidant and is essential in the synthesis of collagen. Humans, unlike other animals, cannot make vitamin C; we must obtain it from our food. Our bodies can store vitamin C for a certain amount of time, but if we go too long without renewing those stores we develop scurvy, and if untreated this leads to death. It really is an essential vitamin.

Nutritionists recommend a daily vitamin C intake of 100 mg. In a healthful, well-balanced diet, this amount is consumed as part of the normal food intake, and no extra supplementation is required. However, when the body is subject to diseases such as HIT, allergies and chronic inflammation it demands a higher Vitamin C intake—around 1,000 mg per day, divided into doses of about 200 mg. The risk of overdosing on Vitamin C is very low because the kidneys excrete any excess. Doses of up to 5,000 mg per day are fine in the short term. [100]

On the Strictly Low Histamine Diet ascorbic acid powder can be used in cooking, to imitate the tang of lemon juice.

B group vitamins (thiamine, riboflavin, niacin, pantothenic acid, pyridoxine, biotin, folic acid or folate, cyanocobalamin).

The vitamins in the B group play vital roles in cell metabolism. Vitamin B deficiencies can cause serious mental and physical problems.

Optimal levels of B vitamins are necessary to maintain good methylation. Without a good supply of B vitamins methylation starts to fail, and the consequences can be disastrous.

Certain substances in food, such as alcohol, animal protein, saturated fat, sugar and coffee can deplete our B vitamins. It is recommended that people suffering from HIT symptoms ensure they have adequate absorption of B group vitamins.

Vitamin B6 (pyridoxine)

Vitamin B6 is thought to have a positive effect on HIT symptoms, however its effectiveness is not entirely uncontroversial. In 2009, German scientist H. Kofler wrote: 'Vitamin B6 is not a cofactor of DAO support.'

Vitamin B6 also inhibits the body's production of oxalate, a histamine-releasing compound which does not appear to be necessary for any human body process and which contribute to the formation of kidney stones.

Methylated Vitamin B12 (methylcobalamin)

Vitamin B12 (cobalamin) is depleted when we take antihistamine drugs for prolonged periods. Additionally, patients with gastric reflux (which is linked to histamine)can be deficient in vitamin B12 after long-term use of proton-pump inhibitors and H2-receptor antagonists (antihistamines) such as cimetidine. Egg yolks, liver, oily fish and meat are the chief dietary sources of vitamin B12.

People with HIT who also have under-methylation are unable to properly absorb B12, which causes problems. These patients should avoid taking standard Vitamin B12 supplements or foods high in B12. For best absorption into the body, it is strongly recommended that Vitamin B12 be consumed in methylated form. Methyl B12 is readily available from alternative therapists and health food stores.

Methylated Folic Acid (methylfolate)

Folate, or folic acid, is a B-group vitamin. Its name comes from the same source as 'foliage', because it occurs in large amounts in leafy dark-green vegetables such as bok choy, Swiss chard and watercress. Taking H2 receptor antihistamines such as Cimetidine lowers folate absorption. [103]

An increased intake of folate is especially important for those who suffer from under-methylation. On the other hand, folate is known to actually raise histamine levels unless it is consumed in the form of methylfolate.

Copper and zinc

Studies on animals have shown that a deficiency in copper is associated with low DAO enzyme activity. [112]

Other research has shown that taking copper supplements significantly increased the activities of DAO in some copper-deficient adult men, although more research is needed. [113]

Zinc can inhibit the release of histamine. [121]

Calcium and vitamin D

Calcium plays a role in the regulation of histamine release. [122] If you are not receiving at least 10 minutes' worth of sunlight on your skin each day, due to seasonal factors or lifestyle, consider taking a vitamin D supplement to improve your calcium absorption.

Magnesium

A magnesium deficiency has been shown to liberate histamine in the body. [123] [124]

SUPPLEMENTS: PROBIOTICS AND ENZYMES

Probiotics

It has been suggested that people suffering from HIT would benefit from a daily dose of a broad-spectrum enzyme supplement composed of a wide range of proteases (enzymes that break down proteins).

Encouraging evidence shows that probiotics are able to mitigate allergic disorders. These beneficial bacterial organisms have many ways of helping our bodies to good health.

Lactobacillus reuteri is a probiotic which uses histamine to actually inhibit tumor necrosis factor (TNF), which is part of the inflammatory response. In other words, it helps to suppress inflammation in the gut. [125]

Research demonstrates, too, that the probiotic Lactobacillus rhamnosus decreases the switching on of H4 receptors and mast cells. Thus, probiotics have the ability to redirect immune responses away from the type of reactions characteristic of histamine functions in autoimmune diseases, allergies and asthma. [126]

It is suggested that combining four strains of probiotics—L. reuteri, L. rhamnosus, L. casei, and B. bifidum—may produce optimum reduction of the allergic reactions that may precipitate histamine overloads. [127]

Enzymes

Bromelain belongs to a group of protein-digesting enzymes obtained commercially from the fruit or stem of pineapple. It is not an antihistamine as such, but it has many therapeutic benefits including anti-inflammatory properties. [96]

Some alternative medicine practitioners recommend that bromelain be taken as an alternative to antihistamines, in conjunction with Vitamin C and quercetin. [95]

Diamine oxidase (DAO) As discussed above, this enzyme breaks down histamine.

People who are deficient in the enzyme diamine oxidase (DAO) may help prevent symptoms by taking DAO-containing products such as DAOsin® or Histame®. Both are manufactured from an extract of pigs' kidneys, which means they are not appropriate for vegetarians. These drugs should be taken 15-30 minutes before meals to ensure distribution of the enzyme along the digestive tract. In this way, much of the histamine in the food you eat may be broken down in the intestines instead of passing into the bloodstream.

While taking DAO supplements may be useful for some, these are not wonder drugs. They only work if you take them before a meal. If you suffer from histamine overload symptoms after a meal, taking DAO supplements will not help. The drugs have other limitations, too: they are also effective only against histamine in the food you eat. They are ineffective against histamine released from mast cells, triggered by histamine liberators, allergens etc.

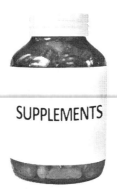

SUPPLEMENTS

SUPPLEMENTS: FLAVONOIDS AND PROPOLIS

Flavonoids (also called bioflavonoids), especially quercetin.

Antioxidant and anti-inflammatory

Flavonoids, whose name derives from the Latin word 'flavus' meaning 'yellow', are colored substances found in plants.

Flavonoids have antioxidant properties, which means that they forage for 'free radicals' (harmful particles) in the body. These free radicals injure cell membranes, meddle with our DNA and even kill cells. Antioxidants can negate free radicals and may decrease or avert their destructive consequences. Additionally, they help prevent artery-clogging LDL cholesterol from being oxidized. Researchers believe this may help to prevent heart disease. Excessive histamine release can be minimized by the use of antioxidants. Flavonoids have also been shown to have valuable anti-inflammatory mechanisms.

Vitamin C and flavonoids

Modern studies have shown that there is a two-way, beneficial relationship between vitamin C and flavonoids. Each compound enhances the antioxidant properties of the other. Furthermore, it seems that numerous functions of vitamin C can only take place in the presence of flavonoids.

Flavonoids inhibit histamine release

At least six flavonoids—fisetin, kaempferol, myricetin, quercetin and rutin—inhibit histamine release. [128]

Foods rich in flavonoids

Foods with abundant flavonoids include broccoli, Brussels sprouts, mangos, persimmons, asparagus and garlic.

Luteolin

The flavonoid luteolin has been shown to inhibit mast cell activity. [129] Dietary sources of luteolin include celery, broccoli, pomegranate, green pepper, parsley, thyme, dandelion, perilla, carrots, olive oil, peppermint, rosemary and oregano. [130]

Quercetin

Quercetin is another flavonoid. It has been shown, in laboratory tests, to help stabilize mast cells and to possess excellent antioxidant and anti-inflammatory characteristics, which may relieve the symptoms of allergies. [162] It is also thought to be anti-viral.

'In test tubes, quercetin prevents immune cells from releasing histamines, chemicals that cause allergic reactions. On that basis, researchers think that quercetin may help reduce symptoms of allergies, including runny nose, watery eyes, hives, and swelling of the face and lips. However, there is no evidence yet that it works in humans.' [167]

Numerous researchers are investigating quercetin for a vast array of potential health treatments, including treatments for chronic prostatitis, high blood pressure and fibromyalgia. [164]

Asthma: Quercetin is an effective bronchodilator and helps decrease the release of histamine and other allergic or inflammatory compounds in the body. [131]

Eczema: Nearly all eczema patients test positive for allergies. Their immunoglobulin E (IgE) levels are generally high. Allergic reactions are caused by the body's release of specific IgE antibodies directed against invading allergens. Quercetin reduces high immunoglobulin E (IgE) levels in the blood of laboratory animals. [161] [133]

Dermatitis: In human test subjects, quercetin effectively blocked histamine release from human mast cells, thus inhibiting contact dermatitis and sensitivity to sunlight. [163]

Hayfever: Other studies demonstrate that quercetin can alleviate symptoms of pollinosis (hayfever). [165]

Cancer: 'Quercetin also displays unique anticancer properties. ... Quercetin is a safe, natural therapy that may be used as
primary therapy or in conjunction with conventional methods.'
[166]

Foods rich in quercetin include onions, raw capers, apples
and leafy green vegetables such as sorrel and lovage.

Propolis

'Propolis is a resinous, strongly adhesive natural substance,
collected by honeybees from the buds and leaves of trees and
plants, and mixed with products of their salivary glands and wax.'
[153]

It is believed that propolis's antibiotic and antifungal properties stop diseases and parasites from invading the hive, and hinder
the growth of pathogenic fungi and bacteria.

The chemical composition of propolis is extremely complex.
More than 200 compounds have been identified. [154] [155]

Many biomedical researchers are focusing their attention on
propolis. Some of their preliminary findings include:

Antimicrobial activity: Introductory laboratory research
indicates that some types of propolis possess antibacterial [168]
and antifungal [169] properties.

Emollient properties: Introductory laboratory research with
animals indicates that propolis may be effective in treating the
inflammatory component of skin and esophageal burns. [170]
[171]

Immunomodulating properties: Researchers record that
propolis exhibits both immunosuppressive and immunostimu-
lant effects [172] [173]. More research is required to determine
whether there is any practical application for these apparently
contradictory pharmacological effects.

Allergy treatment: In people who are sensitive to bees or bee products, propolis can trigger extreme allergic reactions. Nonetheless, laboratory studies on rats have shown that 'propolis may be effective in the relief of symptoms of allergic rhinitis through inhibition of histamine release.' [174] In other studies, propolis has been shown to have a stabilizing effect on mast cells. [175] [176]

Oral hygiene treatment: Propolis may protect against dental caries and other forms of oral disease, due to its antimicrobial properties. [177] [178] [179]

Antioxidant activity: Several studies have documented and examined the antioxidant properties of propolis [180] [181] [182].

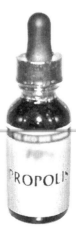

SUPPLEMENTS: HERBS

Albizzia lebbeck—also known as Pit Shirish, Siris Tree, Sharee Tree, Rattle Pod and Women's Tongue.

The leaves, flowers, bark and seed pods are used in traditional medicine on the Indian subcontinent. The leaves are pounded into a paste, which is used as a treatment for skin disorders and to refine skin texture. Paste remedies made from various other parts of the tree are administered to the site of injuries such as bites, cuts and stings. The paste is believed to stimulate healthy teeth and gums, to reduce inflammation. Traditional healers use a powder derived from the tree's leaves, flowers and seed-pods to purify the blood, treat allergies and heal the respiratory system.

Albizzia exhibits a significant antihistamine action. It stabilizes mast cell activity in rats [137]. In animals, Albizzia lebbeck exhibits marked protection against histamine-induced bronchospasm (a sudden constriction of the muscles in the airway).

Tests on animals show that it also has a powerful and almost immediate protective effect against asthma, which can linger (dwindling) for about 24 hours. In human asthma patients, it provided significant relief.

Albizzia lebbeck has been shown to have anti-asthmatic and anti-anaphylactic properties. An orally-administered decoction[1] of the bark and flower of Albizzia lebbeck protects against histamine and broncho-spasm. The drug inhibits the rate at which mast cells are disrupted by allergens.[138]

Furthermore, it protects against histamine in the adrenal glands. [139] [140]

Scutellaria baicalensis—also known as Baikal Skullcap, Blue Skullcap Asian Skullcap or huáng qín.

---

1   To make a decoction, first mash and then boil the plant material in water, to extract oils, volatile organic compounds and other chemical substances. The result is a liquid tea, or tisane.

This is another herb that exhibits a marked antihistamine effect. Note: it is a different species from Scutellaria lateriflora, a Skullcap native to North America.

The plant, which reaches a height between 30 cm (1 foot) and 120cm (4 feet), thrives in sunny spaces on well-drained, poor soils as often occur on grassy mountain slopes. Its leaves are lance-shaped and its tubular, lipped flowers are bluish-purple.

This herb, which is native to Korea, China, Russia, Japan and Mongolia, is one of the 50 fundamental herbs used in traditional Chinese medicine. It has been used for centuries as a remedy for a broad spectrum of inflammatory, allergic and other disorders including diarrhea and other gastrointestinal problems, eczema, hayfever, coughs, fevers, urinary diseases and wheezing. The herb exhibits antioxidant, anti-inflammatory and sedative action, and is a powerful antihistamine. [141]

Baicalein, a compound that occurs in Scutellaria baicalensis has been shown to impede the degranulation of human mast cells and the release of inflammatory cytokines. [142]

Scutellarein, another compound found in this herb, is a potent antiallergic and low cytotoxic flavonoid.

The only part of the plant that is used medicinally is the root, which is harvested when the plant is three to four years old. It is usually processed into either a decoction (tea) or a tincture. Skullcap Tea is used in traditional medicine to treat feverish chest colds, and is taken three times a day.

Tincture of skullcap is made by soaking the root in alcohol. The alcohol acts as a solvent to draw out the herb's useful compounds. As a remedy for allergies, approximately 40 drops of the tincture is mixed with to water and taken thrice daily.

Scutellaria baicalensis is readily available over the counter at pharmacies or health food shops, in stabilized, standardized capsule or tablet form. [141]

Perilla frutescens—also known as Perilla leaf and Shiso. **Carthamus tinctorius**—Safflower leaf.

Scutellarein, the powerful antiallergenic agent and flavonoid found in Baikal Skullcap, has also been detected in perilla leaf and safflower tea infusions. [152]

Plantago major—Common Plantain

Clinical trials have demonstrated that Plantago major is effective in decreasing histamine levels. [143]

This herb also has numerous other benefits. 'Plantago major leaves have been used as a wound healing remedy for centuries in almost all parts of the world and in the treatment of a number of diseases ... A range of biological activities has been found ... including wound healing activity, anti-inflammatory, analgesic, antioxidant, weak antibiotic, immuno modulating and antiulcerogenic activity. Some of these effects may attribute to the use of this plant in folk medicine.' [144]

Rhodiola quadrifida (Chinese common name: si lie hong jing tian, Japanese common name: Shiretsukoukeiten)

Rhodiola quadrifida roots and rhizomes are traditionally used in Asia as a tonic, adaptogen, antidepressant and anti-inflammatory drug. This herb is native to the Jargalant mountain in the western part of Mongolia. After being collected, the roots are air-dried and powdered. They are usually made into a tincture for medicinal purposes. The bioactive constituents of this herb inhibit histamine release and show antiallergic activity [145] [146].

Warning: People with high blood pressure should not take Rhodiola quadrifida.

Rhodiola rosea (commonly known as Golden Root, Rose Root, Roseroot, Aaron's Rod, Arctic Root, King's Crown, Lignum Rhodium, Orpin Rose).

Rhodiola rosea has been shown to have anti-inflammatory properties [147]. It also protects against neurotoxicity, and may help provide a future treatment for neurodegenerative diseases.

Ribes nigrum—Blackcurrant

Blackcurrant seed oil has been shown to be useful in the treatment of atopic dermatitis in dogs. [149] Compounds in the leaves have anti-inflammatory properties. [150] Use externally and do not consume it.

Glycyrrhiza glabra—Licorice

The main ingredient of licorice is 'glycyrrhizin'. Glycyrrhiza glabra has been found to have significant anti-bacterial and anti-oxidant activity. [151]

Saiboku-to

Saiboku-to is a Japanese herbal formula that has been approved by the Japanese Health Ministry for the treatment of asthma. It decreases asthmatic inflammation in numerous trials as compared to placebo.

Saiboku-to contains bupleurum (Bupleurum chinense), hoelen (poria mushroom: Wolfiporia extensa), pinellia (Pinellia ternata—a toxic herb, be warned), magnolia, Asian ginseng (Panax ginseng), Baical Skullcap (Scutellaria baicalensis), licorice ((Glycyrrhiza glabra), perilla (Perilla frutescens), ginger (Zingiber officinale) and jujube(Ziziphus jujuba). [156]

The combination of herbs is thought to have significant anti-inflammatory and antihistamine effects. [157]

Note: Saiboku-to only has efficacy if it is made up by accredited health care professionals, according to the precise, traditional formula, and administered in the correct dose. In any other form it may be dangerous to your health.

MEDICATIONS

Mast cell stabilizers

Mast cell stabilizers are a group of drugs with antiallergic activity. They stabilize the cell membrane of mast cells. This prevents the degranulation of the mast cells and the release of histamine and other (inflammatory) mediators. In the form of eye drops and nasal sprays, mast cell stabilizers are chiefly used to treat pollen allergy. Mast cell stabilizers can help prevent allergic reactions from occurring when they are used regularly.

Quercetin and cromolyn sodium are examples of mast cell stabilizers derived from natural plant extracts.

'As inhalers they are used to treat asthma, as nasal sprays to treat hay fever (allergic rhinitis) and as eye drops for allergic conjunctivitis. In oral form they are used to treat ... mastocytosis.' [158]

Antihistamines (also known as histamine antagonists, histamine receptor blockers or histamine receptor antagonists).

As explained earlier in this book, histamine is a chemical messenger that exerts its effect by targeting various histamine receptors, much like a key that fits into certain locks, whereby it can set a specific mechanism in motion. Antihistamines act against histamine-induced symptoms by blocking specific histamine receptors. Figuratively speaking, they clog certain key holes, so that the key no longer fits. Antihistamines do not act directly against histamine, but they can temporarily block certain effects of histamine.

The four histamine receptors are denoted by H1 to H4. The H1-antihistamines (such as Cetirizine and Loratadine) can usually suppress most allergy symptoms (see glossary). The H2-antihistamines (such as ranitidine and cimetidine) are useful in cases of excessive stomach acid production, with symptoms including heartburn and acid reflux. H3 and H4 blockers currently have no therapeutic significance.

The older antihistamines (known as 'first generation' antihistamines) have the ability to cross the blood-brain barrier. In the brain, they may have a sedative effect on the central nervous system; that is, they can make you tired. During the day, this may be an undesirable side effect. Other adverse reactions can include insomnia and confusion.

Newly developed antihistamines—the 'second generation'— were designed so that they cannot or can only slightly penetrate the blood-brain barrier. Since they cannot reach the central nervous system, they do not cause fatigue. They may, nonetheless, cause headaches and dry mucous membranes.

Examples of second-generation antihistamines include Cetirizine, Desloratadine, Fexofenadine, Loratadine and Levocetirizine.

Why not simply take antihistamines and continue eating foods high in histamine?

Firstly, because antihistamines only target specific receptors. Secondly, because these drugs cannot affect the histamine we consume in foods; they only block histamine from being produced in the body. Thirdly, antihistamines actually shut down the body's security systems. You may have a symptom such as hayfever, which you want to suppress; however by taking an antihistamine you are shutting down defense systems all over your body, not simply in your watery eyes and runny, sneezing nose. Antihistamines do not treat the cause of the symptoms; that is not their purpose. They afford temporary relief by blocking histamine receptors to help us sleep, heal, and battle inflammation. Antihistamines do not improve DAO enzyme activity and long-term use of these drugs is linked with weight gain.

Corticosteroids

Corticosteroid medications — including cortisone, hydrocortisone and prednisone — are widely employed to treat a variety of conditions, from rashes to asthma.

These drugs imitate the activities of the hormones produced naturally in the body. When administered in doses that exceed your body's normal levels, corticosteroids inhibit inflammation, thereby decreasing the symptoms of inflammatory diseases such as asthma, or inflammation triggered by allergens.

Corticosteroids also depress the immune system, which may help to ameliorate auto-immune diseases.

Corticosteroid ointments and creams may be used for a variety of skin allergy conditions, including eczema or atopic dermatitis.

Nasal sprays may contain corticosteroids to reduce swelling and inflammation in nasal passages. Many ointments and creams used to treat skin allergies also contain corticosteroids. In severe cases, these medications may also be administered orally or by injection.

Hydrocortisone, which is is a mild corticosteroid, is prescribed to treat a range of skin conditions including insect bites, eczema, dermatitis, allergies and rashes. It decreases symptoms such as redness, swelling and itching.

Corticosteroids can be purchased in many forms—as tablets or fluids for severe allergies or asthma, as inhalers for asthma, as nasal sprays for hayfever, as topical creams for skin allergies or as eye drops for allergic conjunctivitis.

Side effects and risks exist, in particular when corticosteroids are used long-term or when they are taken by mouth or by injection.

The potential side-effects of short-term use include high blood pressure, fluid retention and weight gain.

With long-term use there is an increased risk of diabetes, osteoporosis, growth suppression in children and adolescents, cataracts of the eyes and muscle weakness.

'Oral use of cortisone has a number of potential systemic side-effects: hyperglycemia, insulin resistance, diabetes mellitus, osteoporosis, anxiety, depression, amenorrhea, cataracts and glaucoma, among other problems.' [159] [160]

7. About the Food List

WHY LISTS OF HISTAMINE LEVELS IN FOOD VARY

Looking through and comparing lists of food histamine levels can be very confusing. Most histamine lists differ from each other, because histamine levels in foods are subject to fluctuation, depending on factors such as the length of time the food has been in storage, the temperature at which food is stored, and the time that has elapsed between when an animal is killed and when it is gutted. A particular fish may have low levels of histamine when it is fresh, higher levels an hour later and even higher levels three hours later. This is in contrast to the measurement of, for example lactose or gluten, which remain constant in spite of storage conditions. Tables of histamine levels are useful, but it must be remembered that they can never be precise and must only suffice as reference points.

Many histamine lists do not take into account foods that may be DAO blockers. Moreover, they may not include mention of oxalate (oxalic acid), an irritant that can trigger histamine release, thereby causing the same symptoms as histamine. Oxalates can also contribute to the distress and debility of chronic fatigue syndrome and myalgic encephalomyelitis, because they damage and destroy mitochondria. High levels of oxalate in the intestines also hinder beneficial bacteria from colonizing the gut.

Nor do many food histamine lists consider foods that release other biogenic amines, those which may contribute to HIT and which certain foods may release in some individuals, despite the fact that the foods themselves may not contain any biogenic amines. [19]

ABOUT THE FOODS LISTED IN THE 'STRICTLY LOW-HISTAMINE' DIET

For the purposes of this book, a number of respected low-histamine food lists were compared, side by side. Our sources included Dr. Janice Joneja Ph.D., RD., Allergy UK, The Swiss Allergy Centre and The Swiss Interest Group Histamine Intolerance (SIGHI).

'Dr. Joneja is a researcher, educator, author, and clinical counselor with over thirty years of experience in the area of biochemical and immunological reactions involved in food allergy and intolerances. She holds a Ph.D. in medical microbiology and immunology, and has been a member of the academic faculty of the University of British Columbia and other universities.

'Dr. Joneja is also a registered dietitian (RD) in the College of Dietitians of British Columbia, a member of Dietitians of Canada, and the American Dietetic Association. For 12 years she was head of the Allergy Nutrition Program at the Vancouver Hospital and Health Sciences Center.

'She is the author of seven books on the immunology of allergy, food allergies and intolerances, and digestive tract reactions to foods. Three of these are peer-reviewed textbooks. Her work has been published in peer-reviewed scientific and medical journals, as well as in popular magazines. Dr. Joneja is a respected lecturer at universities, colleges and hospitals internationally, and regularly appears on television and radio call-in shows as an expert in her field.' [183]

Allergy UK is 'the leading national charity dedicated to supporting the estimated 21 million allergy sufferers in the UK. We provide a dedicated helpline, support network and online forum for those with allergy and intolerance. We also help and support to educate health care professionals who work with patients with allergic conditions.' [184]

The Swiss Allergy Centre is situated in Bern, Switzerland. Its Scientific Advisory Board includes leaders from the field of medical science.

'Swiss Allergy Centre is a non-profit foundation that is active throughout Switzerland, recognized by ZEWO and ISO-certified. We are the centre of excellence in the allergy field and focus on the reactions of the airways, digestive system and skin to environmental irritants. We have a visible public presence as the Swiss Allergy Centre and we are an independent contact point for sufferers and carers, but also for other interested groups such as the media, companies, training centres, politics, authorities and associations. The services we offer range from advising individuals and training courses through to prevention projects and campaigns for the population at large. These offerings are made possible by our widespread network and close cooperation with leading experts and professional bodies in the relevant spheres.'

The Swiss Interest Group Histamine Intolerance (SIGHI), whose website is edited by a small group of authors, which consists of HIT-affected people without any medical education, but who have received an award from the Swiss Allergy Centre for their efforts.

HOW THE FOOD LIST WAS COMPILED.

Certain foods were included on some authoritative lists but not on others. Wheat germ was generally considered undesirable, but wheat bran appeared to be permissible.

There was disagreement about the following fruits, vegetables and spices: Cherries, grapes, cranberries, blackberries, peaches, apricots, nectarines, pears, black-currants and red-currants, blueberries, kiwi-fruit, pineapple, plums, papaya, mushrooms, broad beans, pumpkin, anise, cinnamon, nutmeg and cloves.

Legumes and pulses were also debatable. Some lists included non-soy legumes such as dried beans and peas and lentils. All lists banned soy and red beans.

Again, some lists banned all nuts, while others forbade only walnuts, pecans and cashews.

In the end we limited our own list to foods that were accepted as 'low histamine' (in all its senses) by every authority, and about which there was little or no debate. In consequence, our catalogue of acceptable ingredients is restricted, but as 'safe' as possible.

The 'Strictly Low Histamine Diet' omits all foods recognized as containing high levels of histamine or containing chemicals that may boost the release of histamine in the body or inhibit histamine breakdown. It includes food rich in the nutrients our bodies require to combat histamine imbalance. The recipes in Part II combine these nutritious foods in a variety of delicious dishes.

The diet includes seven basic food groups:
* Vegetables
* Fruit
* Dairy Products & Egg Yolks
* Cereals, Grains & Starches
* Fats & Oils
* Spices & Herbs
* Sweeteners

In general, it avoids three other groups; meat and poultry, seafood, and nuts and seeds. However, as you progress and your symptoms fade, you can begin to add certain foods back into your diet, one by one, remembering to ensure that everything you eat is as fresh as possible.

PROTEIN

On the Strictly Low Histamine Diet your protein comes from fresh egg yolks, certain dairy foods and grains (cereals). It resembles a vegetarian diet minus the legumes and pulses.

Food grains (cereals) are rich in carbohydrates, B-vitamins, energy and protein. If they are one of your chief sources of protein, you should choose grains with a high protein to carbohydrate ratio. In general, whole, unrefined grains, supply more protein per carbohydrate.

Durum wheat (used to make pasta) and whole grain wheat flour (used to make bread) contain 1 gram of protein per 5 grams of carbohydrates, but the wheat germ contained in these cereals triggers histamine release, so wheat flour should generally be avoided.

Below is a hierarchy of protein per gram of carbohydrates for low-histamine food grains. If gluten gives you problems, avoid the spelt, barley and rye.

> **Oat bran**—1 gram protein to 3 grams carbs.
> **Rice bran, oats and wheat bran**—1 gram protein to 4 grams carbs.
> **Rye, spelt, wild rice and teff**[2]—1 gram protein to 5 grams carbs.
> **Barley**—1 gram protein to 6 grams carbs.
> **Black rice, sorghum and millet**—1 gram protein to 7 grams carbs.
> **Yellow or white corn**—1 gram protein to 8 grams carbs.
> **Brown rice**—1 gram protein to 9 grams carbs. [193]
> **Water-chestnut flour**—1 gram protein to 17 grams carbs.

---

2   Teff: Eragrostis tef, also known as lovegrass, annual bunch grass, taf, or 'mil éthiopien'—French for 'Ethiopian millet'.

If you intend to follow this diet we advise you to prepare food immediately prior to eating it. Do not consume leftovers, or any dishes prepared on the previous day unless it has been frozen in the interim, to stop histamine levels from rising.

Naturally, if you are allergic to any of these foods you must avoid them.

8. The Strictly Low Histamine Diet

FRESHNESS

The importance of fresh foods for the Strictly Low Histamine Diet cannot be overestimated. We suggest growing your own herbs, fruit and vegetables in your home garden. That way you'll always have a fresh supply of 'live' food.

Even if you don't have a garden, you could try growing potted herbs such as basil, lemon verbena, mint and parsley on a sunny kitchen windowsill or on a balcony.

FOODS TO ENJOY

Vegetables

All vegetables except forbidden ones (see the list "Vegetables to Avoid" on page 88). Permitted vegetables include beetroot; broccoli; cauliflower; zucchini (courgette); cucumber; green beans; lettuce; cabbage; roquette, parsnip; radish; sweet corn; leeks; spirulina (*Arthrospira maxima* and *A. plaetensis*); chinese cabbage; spring onion (scallion); carrot; Brussels sprouts; bok choy; mustard greens; fennel; celery, snap peas; asparagus, and sweet potatoes. Good sources of quercetin include onions, dill, garlic, broccoli and lettuce.

Egg Yolks

Fresh, cooked, free range egg yolks and raw egg yolk can be eaten freely. (Many people can also tolerate cooked egg whites.) Avoid eggs that are not fresh. Choose free range eggs from *pastured* hens, because free-roaming pastured hens have access to a wide assortment of insects, worms and fresh greens, which means their eggs are of much higher nutritional value.

Pastured hens have been found to produce eggs with four times more omega-3s than the eggs of caged hens. The eggs also contain significantly more vitamin E and vitamin A, and less fat.

Caged hens only have access to commercial, manufactured chicken food, which may contain added hormones and antibiotics. Furthermore, caged hens have high levels of stress hormones, which may have a deleterious effect on their eggs.

Fresh Fruit

Apples (a good source of quercetin); melons; watermelon; honeydew melon; rock melon (cantaloupe); mangos; persimmons; figs; passionfruit; pomegranate; rhubarb; starfruit; longans; lychees; quinces; goldenberries[3] (Physalis peruviana); loquats.

Dairy products and milks

Oat milk and rice milk - store-bought or make your own ["A Variety of Milks" on page 94].

Oat cream and rice cream ["A Variety Of Delicious Creams (Non-Dairy)" on page 100]

---

3   This delicious fruit is also known as Cape gooseberry, Inca berry, Aztec berry, giant ground cherry, Peruvian groundcherry, Peruvian cherry and Pichuberry. In temperate climates, it is easily grown in the home garden.

Pure, fresh milk (pasteurized); ricotta and mascarpone with no forbidden additives; pure cream; pure ice-cream; butter; uncultured, plain buttermilk.

Note: Many people avoid dairy products for ethical reasons[4], or because they contain bovine growth hormones, which are thought to be linked to obesity. The casein in dairy foods may cause problems for some people. [186]

Fats and Oils

Vegetable oils, preferably cold-pressed, especially rice bran oil and olive oil; pure butter and cream.

Beverages

Coffee; milk; milkshakes with permitted ingredients; iced water; soda and mineral water; chamomile tea, peppermint tea, dandelion tea, ginger tea, rooibos tea, chicory beverages.

Cereals, Grains, Pseudocereals & Starches

Rice, wild rice, black, red or purple rice, rice bran (especially bran from pigmented rice); pure, unbleached flour blends containing permitted ingredients; crackers without yeast; baked products leavened with baking powder; corn (not canned corn); rye; spelt; millet; teff; oats; oat bran; wheat bran; wheat in small quantities; sorghum; barley, polenta; chia seeds; hemp seeds; sweet chestnuts (*Castanea sativa*). If for any reason you cannot avoid eating eat wheat bread, choose wholemeal.

4　Calves born on dairy farms are taken from their mothers when they are one day old and fed milk replacements so that the mothers' milk can be sold for use by humans. The mothers can be heard calling for their babies for up to several weeks. On average an equal number of male and female calves are born to dairy cows. Male calves are usually killed when they are about five days old. Cows stop producing milk unless they give birth every year.

Baking Agents and Starches:

Guar gum; agar agar; baking powder; baking soda.

Cornstarch/cornflour; arrowroot; sago[5] flour/sago starch; rice flour; water-chestnut flour (Eleocharis dulcis); potato flour; potato starch[6].

Sweet rice flour can also be used in baking, but it is rather adhesive and viscous, so be sparing and use no more than ¼ cup in your recipe or you might end up with a sticky, glutinous end product.

Spices, Herbs, Flavorings & Condiments

Permitted condiments include salt, black or white pepper, fresh curry leaves and wasabi.

All fresh, frozen, or dried herbs and spices are allowed, *except* those on the 'restricted' list. Use fresh herbs, and preferably grind your own spice seeds.

Permitted herbs and spices include turmeric; sumac; cardamom; allspice; asafoetida; ginger root; tarragon; bay leaf; pimento leaf; basil; parsley; rosemary; garlic; galangal; mint; chocolate mint; peppermint; oregano; chives; sage; culinary myrtle leaf, fenugreek; savory; marjoram; caraway and coriander (cilantro) [190]. Dill is particularly high in quercetin.

Pure pomegranate molasses is a wonderful seasoning and citrus replacement. A recipe for pomegranate molasses can be found in the chapter entitled 'Sauces and Condiments'.

---

5   See glossary

6   Note: Potato flour is not identical to potato starch. Potato flour is heavy and sticky, not much use in baking but good for thickening sauces and gravies. Potato starch, on the other hand, makes delicate, elastic breads, cakes and muffins. Also potatoes contain oxalates, which can release histamine in some people.

Amchoor is dried sour mango powder. [Recipe on page 114] It can also be made from tart apples. Ascorbic acid powder, mango amchoor or apple amchoor can be used as a substitute for lemon juice.

You can use black cumin seeds, but not ordinary cumin. 'Black cumin' may refer to the seeds of *Bunium bulbocastanum* or *Nigella sativa*. Both have antihistamine properties and can be used.

Note: parsley and chives are relatively high in oxalates, so use them sparingly.

All artificial essences and flavoring extracts are banned. Natural, pure vanilla extract or essence is not permitted if it contains alcohol.

Natural, oil-based, alcohol-free vanilla, caramel, rose, cardamom, lavender, violet and peppermint extracts are permitted; also natural coffee essence. Somewhat more exotic flavors include Khus extract—from vetiver grass (*Chrysopogon zizanioides*) and edible Kewra oil (Attar of Kewra)—a concentrated oil made from the flowers of pandan (*Pandanus odoratissimus*).

Large supermarkets generally stock edible essential oils near the spice department. They may also be bought in cake and candy supply stores or pharmacies, and in general they can be stored indefinitely in a cool, dark place.

Edible essential oils are usually stronger than flavoring extracts. In recipes, four parts of flavoring extract is roughly equivalent to one part of flavoring oil, but this may vary according to the brand.

Natural colorings that can be made at home or store-bought include:

BROWN: caramel coloring made from caramelized sugar, ["Caramel Essence" on page 128] and coffee essence, ["Coffee Essences" on page 123]

RED: pure cochineal (*not* 'cochineal coloring'), red cabbage juice and beetroot juice

MAGENTA: purple cabbage juice and the juice of the Magenta Plant (*Peristrophe roxburghiana*), which easily grown in frost-free gardens

ORANGE/YELLOW: turmeric and saffron

GREEN: pandan (*Pandanus amaryllifolius*)

BLACK: ramie (*Boehmeria nivea*)

BLUE: butterfly pea (*Clitoria ternatea*)

Sweeteners

Pasteurized honey[7]; white sugar; brown sugar; icing (confectioners') sugar; maple syrup; corn syrup; brown rice syrup; agave nectar; treacle; golden syrup; brown rice syrup; molasses; jaggery; palm sugar; pure jams and jellies; marmalade; conserves made with allowed ingredients; plain artificial sweeteners.

Legumes, Pulses, Nuts & Seeds

Avoid all.

---

7   Infants, people with HIT and people with compromised immune systems should consume only pasteurized honey. Unpasteurized honey has a very small chance of containing spores of the pathogen Clostridium botulinum, which is harmless to healthy adults but may cause problems for people with HIT.

Special antihistamine foods

These include black rice, black rice bran, red or purple rice and ascorbic acid powder.

Onions, garlic, apples, parsley, broccoli and lettuce are good sources of quercetin.

SUPPLEMENTS

If you believe you are not receiving enough nourishment from food, or if your symptoms are severe, you may wish to supplement your diet.

Recommended supplements include vitamin C, vitamin B (preferably methylated, especially B12, B6 and folate), vitamin E, propolis (if you are not sensitive to bee products), probiotics (especially L. reuteri, L. rhamnosus, L. casei, and B. bifidum), quercetin, bromelain, copper, zinc, calcium and magnesium.

We do, however, reiterate that nutrition from real food is generally better balanced and absorbed than nutrition from man-made supplements.

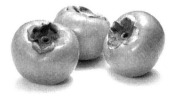

FOODS TO AVOID

Vegetables

Overripe or rotten vegetables; tomatoes; raw onion; buckwheat; all fermented vegetables, such as sauerkraut; all pickled vegetables; spinach; eggplant; avocado; packaged salad mixes; packaged peeled vegetables; bell peppers (capsicum); fermented soy products; purslane, pumpkin. Winter squash is closely related to pumpkin, so to be on the safe side we do not recommend it. Note that kale is high in oxalates, which are irritants that may cause histamine release, so it's best to avoid it.

Fruit

Strawberries; citrus fruits; all berries and stone fruits; raisins and sultanas; papayas; bananas; pineapple; dates; avocados; pears; coconut, any dried fruit preserved with sulfur; overripe or rotten fruit.

Dairy Products & Eggs

Yoghurt; all cheeses except fresh mascarpone, quark and ricotta; unpasteurized milk; cultured buttermilk, cultured cream, sour cream, stale eggs, raw egg white (such as is sometimes used in sorbet).

Cereals, Grains & Starches

Buckwheat; quinoa; yeast; baked goods made with yeast; wheat germ; amaranth (it's high in oxalates).
Baking agents & starches
Xanthan gum; gelatin; carrageenan; tapioca starch[8] (also known as tapioca flour or cassava starch).

---

8   Cassava is high in oxalates.

Legumes, Pulses, Nuts and Seeds

All legumes, pulses, nuts and seeds including walnuts, pecans, cashews and sesame seeds. Anything made with soy.

Fats and Oils

Margarine, avocado flesh, coconut oil and coconut cream.

Spices, Herbs, Flavorings and Condiments

Artificial flavors; alcohol-based flavors; anise; cinnamon; nutmeg and mace; cloves; chocolate; cocoa; thyme; chili; curry; hot/spicy seasonings; mustard seed; smoke flavor; soy sauce; tamari; soy products; brewer's yeast; tamarind (because it is usually fermented); cayenne pepper; any foods containing vinegar.

Sweeteners

Flavored syrups; prepared dessert fillings; prepared icings/frostings; spreads with restricted ingredients; cake decorations; commercial confectionery and candies; unpasteurized honey.

Beverages

Soft drinks; alcohol in general, particularly red wine and beer; black tea; green tea; red raspberry tea; maté tea; energy drinks.

Meat, Poultry & Seafood

All meat, poultry and seafood (fish, octopus, shellfish etc.), but especially processed meat such as sausage, bratwurst, cabana, smoked salmon etc. Leftovers, especially high protein leftovers.

~ PART II: RECIPES ~

MEASUREMENTS

All measurements are metric, with avoirdupois equivalents in brackets. All cup measurements are 250 ml.

The U.S. cup is 240 ml, close enough to do a cup to cup conversion except in baking recipes in which accuracy is critical.

The U.K. cup is 225ml, which is sufficient difference for cooks to do conversion calculations when baking. There are many free measurement conversion websites online.

GLUTEN

Gluten free recipes are marked with [GF]. Gluten is only a problem for people who have been diagnosed with celiac disease (approximately 1% of the population), or who are non-celiac gluten sensitive (NCGS), a condition that is distinct from celiac disease.

In these people, eating gluten can lead to 'leaky gut' syndrome and thence to DAO insufficiency and histamine intolerance.

If you are, like most people, capable of digesting gluten without any problems, gluten-containing foods are good for you. They are highly nutritious—packed with vitamins, minerals and beneficial fiber.

All people who suffer from histamine intolerance should, however, avoid eating wheat germ.

9. Basic Recipes, Substitutes and Hints

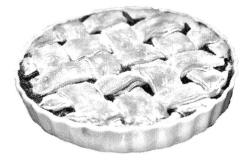

A VARIETY OF MILKS

Oat milk, rice milk and uncultured buttermilk are available at many supermarkets. However if you cannot obtain them or if you avoid the additives in commercial products, here's how to make them at home.

[GF] QUICK OAT MILK

This quick and easy recipe yields a milk that is rather thinner than 'Slow Oat Milk'. It can be thickened by either the addition of a little finely ground oat bran, or by cooking the rolled oats before you make the milk.

---

1 cup rolled oats
water for soaking
3 cups water
sweetener of your choice (optional)
ground cardamom or allspice (optional)
natural caramel essence (optional)

Note: you will also need a blender and a fine sieve or cheese cloth.

Put the oats in a large bowl and add enough water to just cover them. Allow to rest for 10 minutes.

Drain the oats and pour into blender. Add 3 cups of water and sweetener or additional flavorings if desired. If you wish, you may add more or less water, depending on the consistency you prefer.

Blend until the oats have completely disintegrated into a creamy liquid.

Strain the milk through a fine sieve or cheese cloth (this is optional). Homemade oat milk keeps for a few days under refrigeration, but while standing it may separate, so make sure you shake or stir it before using.

[GF] SLOW OAT MILK

> 1 cup steel-cut oats
> 3 cups water
> 1.5 - 2 tablespoon liquid sweetener of your choice (optional)
> ½ - 1 teaspoon natural oil-based vanilla extract (optional)
> scant ¼ teaspoon salt
> ¼ teaspoon ground cardamom or allspice (optional)

Rinse and drain the oats. Place them into a bowl, cover with water and soak for a minimum of 20 minutes.

Drain and thoroughly rinse the oats. Pour them into a blender and add 3 cups water. For a thinner consistency, add more water.

Process at a low speed, gradually increasing the speed, and blend at the highest speed for no more than 8-10 seconds.

Put a fine-meshed sieve over a large bowl and strain the oat milk very slowly.

Use a large spoon to gently push down on the oat pulp and squeeze out as much milk as possible.

Place the oat pulp into a small bowl and set it aside. Wash all pulp residue from blender and sieve.

Put clean sieve on top of blender and strain the milk through.

Optionally, you can rinse oat residue from the bowl and sieve and strain the oat milk a third time.

Beat in the flavorings—liquid sweetener, extract, salt and spice. If you wish to use the milk in a savory dish, omit these.

Strain the milk for a fourth time (optional) into a clean vessel with a lid, seal the container and store it in the fridge.

Basic Slow Oat milk should last for 4-5 days. Homemade oat milk separates while standing, so make sure you shake or stir it before using.

[GF] BROWN RICE MILK

¾ **cup brown rice**
3 cups of water
4 ½ cups of extra water
½ teaspoon natural oil-based vanilla extract

Place rice and 3 cups of water in a saucepan and bring them to a boil.

Reduce heat to low and simmer for 45 minutes, adding water if the mixture becomes dry.

When rice is tender, remove it from heat and add 4 ½ extra cups of water and the extract. Stir, then allow to rest for 45 minutes.

Pour the mixture into a blender or food processor, and process for 3-4 minutes.

Strain through a fine sieve or cheese cloth into a clean container with a lid.

Store in the refrigerator. Will keep for 4-5 days.

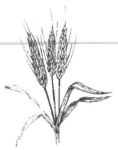

ABOUT BUTTERMILK

In the USA, cultured, thick milk is commonly called 'buttermilk'—however that is something of a misnomer.

True buttermilk is made by churning fresh cream to separate out the fat solids. The result is butter on the one hand, and low-fat milk on the other.

Buttermilk is more easily digestible than whole milk and has less fat. It is also preferred, by many cooks, for baking—especially for pancakes.

People on a low histamine diet should avoid cultured products, but if you cannot buy true buttermilk at your grocery store, what's the solution?

Some cookbooks suggest adding lemon juice or vinegar to regular milk to create buttermilk; however neither of these additives is safe for HIT sufferers.

Another alternative—though a poor one—is to whisk together 1 cup skim milk with 1-¾ tablespoon cream of tartar. Allow the milk to rest at room temperature for 5-10 minutes and stir before you use it. The refined tartaric acid adds a flavor reminiscent of buttermilk and also curdles the milk allowing it to become slightly thicker.

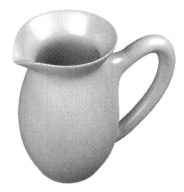

[GF] UNCULTURED DAIRY BUTTERMILK

Here's how to make your own uncultured dairy buttermilk:

> **2 cups of fresh cream**

- Pour 2 cups of fresh dairy cream into the bowl of your food processor (or 4 cups if you have a machine with at least 11-cup capacity). Leave the rest in the refrigerator.
- Begin processing and watch closely as the cream thickens and whips. It may take quite some time. Gradually the cream will start to look less pale. When you see it breaking into tiny yellowish lumps, proceed with caution until you can see that the cream has definitely separated into cloudy buttermilk and clumps of yellow butter.
- Place a strainer over a chilled bowl and pour through the contents of the processor, scraping out any sticky butter particles with a rubber spatula.
- Repeat the entire procedure with the other half of the cream. You now have around 2 cups of buttermilk! Pour the strained buttermilk into a storage container and store it in the refrigerator.

You also have about a cup of unsalted butter. Your strainer will be filled with small lumps of it. Turn the contents out into a bowl and work the butter into one big lump with a strong wooden spoon. Drain off as much liquid as possible and continue working the butter. As the butterfat comes together it will turn into a smooth, shiny mass. When no more liquid emerges, pat the butter dry with paper towels, place it into an airtight container and refrigerate it.

[GF] DAIRY FREE BUTTERMILK

> **1 tablespoon L-ascorbic acid powder or cream of tartar (or less, according to your taste)**
>
> **sufficient non-dairy milk to make up to 1 cup**

- Place L-ascorbic acid powder or cream of tartar in a measuring cup.
- Add enough non-dairy milk of your choosing to make up to one cup. Whisk to combine.
- Allow mixture to rest for 5-10 minutes before using.

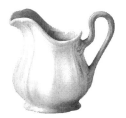

A VARIETY OF DELICIOUS CREAMS (NON-DAIRY)

If you prefer your cream to be free from animal hormones, lower in saturated fats and equally delicious, Oat Cream or Cornstarch Cream may suit you.

Other HIT-friendly creams to choose from include Rice Cream, (as distinct from creamed rice) and HIT-friendly Sour Cream. If you cannot find them in stores, read on...

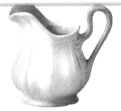

[[GF] MOUTHWATERING WHIPPED RICE CREAM

This is a delicious cream made from rice, not the dish known as 'Creamed Rice'!

Note: In this recipe, standard rice flour cannot be substituted for sweet rice flour. Sweet rice flour, also known as glutinous[9] rice flour sticky rice flour or mochiko, has glue-like characteristics. It is readily available in Asian grocery stores and larger supermarkets.

If you cannot find sweet rice flour, you could either buy sweet rice in grain form and grind it to flour in a powerful food processor, or substitute cornflour (cornstarch).

> **1 cup brown rice milk [page 96]**
> **3 tablespoons sweet rice flour**
> **1 cup non-dairy or dairy butter**
> **1 cup sugar (or sweetener of your choice)**
> **½ teaspoon vanilla extract (optional)**

Place milk and rice flour in a large saucepan (or bowl if you are using a microwave) and cook over a medium heat, stirring frequently, until the mixture becomes very thick. This should take about 5 minutes.

Allow mixture to cool.

Meanwhile, beat together the butter and sugar, continuing to beat until it is no longer grainy. (An electric mixer helps considerably.)

Pour the cooled rice mixture into the creamed butter and sugar, and whip until light and fluffy.

Makes about 4 cups.

---

9   It contains no gluten. 'Glutinous' means 'sticky'.

[GF] CORNSTARCH CREAM

This recipe makes a thick liquid cream, like unwhipped cream. Sweeteners are optional.

> **220 ml (7 fluid ounces) rice milk or other milk [page 313]**
> **3 tablespoons sugar or sweetener of your choice**
> **2 level teaspoons cornflour (cornstarch)**
> **approx. 180 ml (6 fluid ounces) olive oil or rice bran oil**
> **1 teaspoon natural, oil-based vanilla extract (optional)**

Divide the milk into 2 quantities—120 ml (8 tablespoons) and 100 ml (7 tablespoons).

Place in a saucepan the cornstarch and 4 tablespoons of the 120 ml cold milk. Blend them together to form a thin paste, adding a few drop more milk if necessary.

Add the remainder of the 120 ml, then put the saucepan over a low heat and stir the mixture until it thickens.

Pour the thickened milk, the sugar and the vanilla into a blender. Blend at low speed until all ingredients are well mixed, adding the extra 100 ml (7 tablespoons) milk.

Continue to process while gradually adding the vegetable oil.

If the mixture curdles, stop the machine, stir the mixture with a spoon—adding some extra milk if necessary—and keep on blending and pouring in the oil.

Hint: If you'd prefer to make a whippable corn cream, swap the vegetable oil for butter. Melt the butter first and pour it gradually into the running blender, just as you would with the vegetable oil.

To store, chill the cornstarch cream in the refrigerator.

[GF] WHIPPED CORNSTARCH CREAM

> **3 teaspoons cornflour (cornstarch)**
> **1 cup rice milk or milk of your choice [page 80]**
> **4 tablespoons butter, softened [page 85]**
> **4 tablespoons sugar or sweetener of your choice**
> **natural caramel essence**

Put cornstarch and a little of the milk into a saucepan and mix to a smooth paste. Add the rest of the milk, mix well, and set the saucepan on a medium heat.

Bring to the boil, stirring continuously, then turn down the heat to low and simmer for 3 to 4 minutes until the mixture is thick. Stir frequently to keep it from scorching.

Remove from heat and allow to cool.

Place butter and sugar in a chilled mixing bowl and whip until the mixture is well blended and resembles cream.

Slowly add creamed butter and sugar to the cool cornstarch mixture, while beating very thoroughly. Add a couple of drops of extract if desired, and serve.

Store in the refrigerator.

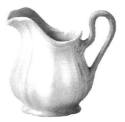

[GF] LUSCIOUS CORNSTARCH CREAM

> **6 egg yolks**
> **½ cup sugar**
> **2 tablespoons flour with permitted ingredients**
> **2 tablespoons cornflour (cornstarch)**
> **2 cups milk of your choice [page 313]**
> **1 teaspoon natural oil-based vanilla essence**
> **(optional)**

Place sugar and egg yolks into a medium sized bowl (this is easier if you use an electric mixer) and beat them until the mixture becomes thick and light.

Gradually add the flour and cornstarch, slowly beating the mixture all the while.

Pour the milk into a saucepan, place it over a medium heat and just bring it barely to a boil, stirring all the while. Then slowly add milk to egg mixture.

Return the mixture to the saucepan. Bring it to a boil again, beating constantly to prevent burning and sticking. When the mixture is thick and pulling away from the sides of the pan, it is ready. This takes 4 to 5 minutes.

Stir in vanilla.

Using a rubber spatula, push mixture through a sieve into a bowl, to remove any lumps. Immediately cover the surface with plastic wrap to stop a 'skin' from forming, place the cream in the refrigerator and let it cool to room temperature.

[GF] OAT CREAM

This recipe is perfect if you are looking for a subtle and mild flavor.

½ cup oat milk
½ cup vegetable oil, such as rice bran oil
1 tablespoon maple syrup
¼ teaspoon natural caramel essence
½ teaspoon agar agar powder (optional for thick-
    ness)
ice (optional)

Place all ingredients in an electric mixer, blender or food processor. Start on low speed and increase to high.

Blend until desired consistency is reached. If serving immediately, add a few ice cubes at the end to counteract heat. Serve chilled.

Store for one week in refrigerator, or freeze 3-6 months.

[GF] HIT-FRIENDLY SOUR CREAM

1 cup unsweetened, whipped HIT-friendly cream
⅓ teaspoon mango amchoor [page 114]
a pinch of salt
1 tablespoon onion powder (optional)

Put all ingredients in blender and process for 2 minutes or until smooth.

A VARIETY OF LOW HISTAMINE REPLACEMENTS

Our Strictly Low Histamine Diet food substitutes are designed to appeal to your palate.

HIT-FRIENDLY 'BACON'

The characteristics of bacon that appeal to most people are smokiness, fat, texture and saltiness. Try grilling some zucchini (courgette) or onions on your barbecue, to add to your fake-bacon recipe.

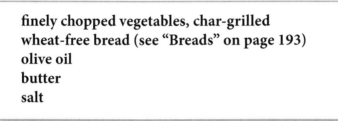

**finely chopped vegetables, char-grilled
wheat-free bread (see "Breads" on page 193)
olive oil
butter
salt**

Use gluten free bread if you wish. Tear the bread into small, irregular pieces. Sauté them in hot olive oil and butter. The wispier parts of will crisp up and start to brown while the thicker bits will absorb the oil.

Next, stir in some generous pinches of salt and the finely chopped char-grilled vegetables. Remove the pan from the heat. Your 'bacon bits' are ready; smoky, salty, crisp and chewy.

Fake bacon bits can be used to garnish vegetable gratins and casseroles. They also make a delicious salad topping.

[GF] LEMON JUICE REPLACEMENT

Citrus, including lemon essence or lemon extract, is not included in the Strictly Low Histamine Diet, yet lemon juice is one of the most versatile and delicious condiments. We can replace it with the juice of green (unripe) mangos ["Green Mango Juice" on page 116] or even with the juice of unripe apples mixed with ascorbic acid powder. Mango or apple amchoor ["Amchoor" on page 114] can also be used in cooking, to replace lemon juice.

[GF] LEMON REPLACEMENTS

The following lemony herbs, fresh, frozen or infused in oils ["Fragrant, Flavored Oils" on page 116], impart a delicious citrus flavor to your recipes:

Lemon Myrtle (Backhousia citriodora)
Lemon Balm (Melissa officinalis)
Lemon Basil (Ocimum xcitriodorum)
Lemon Catmint (Nepeta cataria 'Citriodora')
Lemon Verbena (Aloysia citriodora, Aloysia triphylla)
Lemon Grass (Cymbopogon citratus)
Sumac (Rhus coriaria). The flavor is lemony: tart, sour, fruity, tangy, and zingy.

[GF] LIME REPLACEMENT

Kaffir lime leaves (Citrus hystrix)

[GF] HIT-FRIENDLY 'MUSHROOM'

Cauliflower or zucchini (courgette) can add a mushroom-like texture to dishes. Season it well to compensate for the lack of mushrooms' earthy flavor.

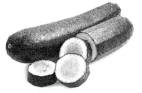

[GF] HIT-FRIENDLY VANILLA ALTERNATIVES

Just for variety, try one of these vanilla extract alternatives. There will of course be changes in flavor, but they will be subtle.

Maple syrup—replace the vanilla with an equal amount of maple syrup.

Natural, oil-based, alcohol-free caramel (or cardamom) essence. Swap the vanilla for an equal quantity of these flavorings.

Molasses, golden syrup, honey, brown rice syrup or treacle may provide an acceptable vanilla substitute.

You might also try our recipes for apple caramel and coffee essence.

[GF] HIT-FRIENDLY CHOCOLATE

To be honest, there is no substitute for chocolate. There are, nonetheless, some foods which, in the absence of the real thing, may help satisfy chocolate cravings.

The **Common Lime** tree (Tilia x europaea), the **Small Leaved Lime** (Tilia cordata) and the **Large Leaved Lime** (Tilia platyphyllos) are mentioned by PFAF[10] as making a good chocolate substitute. (Though called 'lime' trees, these plants are not related to citrus.)

'A very acceptable chocolate substitute can be made from a paste of the ground-up flowers[11] and immature fruit [of lime trees]. Trials on marketing the product failed because the paste is very apt to decompose.' [204][205]

If you have no access to a Lime Tree, you could try the herb **Water Avens** (Geum rivale). This is another chocolate substitute, rated equally with carob for flavor, though not as highly rated as the Lime Tree.

'The dried or fresh root can be boiled in water to make a delicious chocolate-like drink [206][207][208][209][210].

---

10   PFAF: Plants For A Future.
11   Note: If the flowers used ... are too old, they may produce symptoms of narcotic intoxication. [Grieve. A Modern Herbal. 1931]

'It can also be used as a seasoning. It is best harvested in the spring or autumn but can be used all year round. Fragrant, it was once used to flavor ales.'

Carob (Ceratonia siliqua)

The pulp inside the seedpods is sweet and edible. It is dried, roasted and then ground into a cocoa-colored powder which can be used as a chocolate substitute in cakes, drinks etc. It does not, however, have the same texture as chocolate, nor the same flavor.

Chocolate Mint (Mentha × piperita f. citrata 'Chocolate')

Not really a chocolate substitute but a delicious flavoring nonetheless, chocolate mint tastes rather like 'After-Dinner Mints'. The leaves have a chocolate-mint fragrance and can be used in desserts or as a garnish.

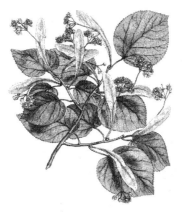

The Lime Tree

HIT-FRIENDLY 'PARMESAN CHEESE'

> **400g (14 ounces) fine, dry, wheat-free**
> **breadcrumbs (see "Breads" on page 193)**
> **½ tablespoon dried basil**
> **½ tablespoon dried oregano**
> **½ tablespoon dried parsley**
> **½ teaspoon salt**
> **⅛ teaspoon dried thyme**
> **⅛ teaspoon dried rosemary**
> **⅛ teaspoon black pepper**
> **2 tablespoons garlic powder**
> **2 tablespoons onion powder**
> **2 tablespoons olive oil or rice bran oil**

Preheat oven to 180°C (350°F)

Spread crumbs in a shallow baking pan and bake in the center of the oven, stirring occasionally, until they turn golden-brown. This should take 10 to 15 minutes.

Mix the other ingredients in a spice grinder, or place into a small bowl and crush with the back of a spoon.

Transfer the toasted crumbs to a bowl, then drizzle with oil and season with herb mixture. Stir until crumbs are coated.

This can be stored in an airtight bag in the freezer for up to 6 months.

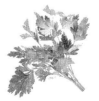

HINT: OIL FOR FRYING

Many people prefer to use non-stick frypans for cooking, so that they do not load up on fats and oils. If, however, you prefer cooking with vegetable oils, choose a high smoke-point oil[12] such as rice bran oil. Oils with a high smoke point are suitable for high-temperature frying (above 230 °C or 446 °F).

Rice bran oil has the added advantages of having a mild flavor and of being extracted from rice bran, which has antihistamine properties.

If using butter for frying, keep temperatures as low as possible.

HINT: HOW TO BLANCH VEGETABLES

To blanch vegetables, make ready a large bowl of ice water, a slotted spoon, and a plate lined with a cloth or paper towel.

Bring a large pot of water to boil over a high heat[13]. Meanwhile, chop your chosen vegetables into uniform pieces, keeping each type of vegetable separate.

Blanch each type of vegetable, beginning with the lighter colored ones. Simply pour the vegetables into the pot in small batches so that the water keeps boiling.

After about a minute, test to see whether the vegetables have reached your preferred consistency. To do this, take the slotted spoon and remove one piece. Dip it into the bowl of ice water, then taste. Keep sampling every 30-60 seconds until the vegetables are cooked to your liking. Most vegetables take 2-5 minutes.

When they are ready, quickly scoop them out of the boiling water with a slotted spoon and drop them into the ice water to halt the cooking process. When cool, drain on the towel-lined plate.

---

12   Oils with a low smoke point degrade easily to toxic compounds when heated. Prolonged consumption of burnt oils may lead to atherosclerosis, inflammatory joint disease, and development of birth defects. [Wikipedia: Cooking oil. Retrieved January 2014]

13   Some people add a pinch of salt to the water to maintain the bright-color of the vegetables; however this leaches nutrients out of the food.

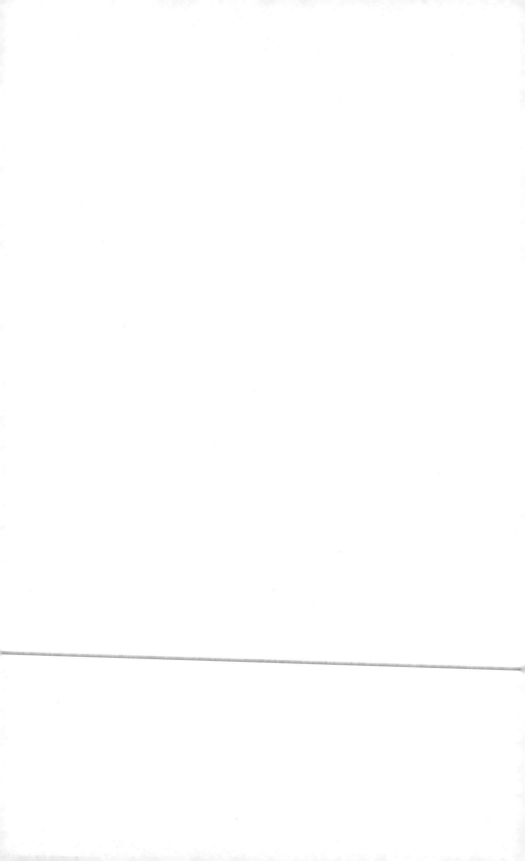

10. Flavorings, Colorings & Seasonings

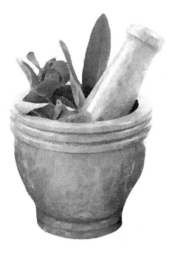

Natural, oil-based, alcohol-free HIT-friendly flavorings such as caramel, vanilla, rose, cardamom, lavender[14], violet, peppermint and coffee essences are available from stores, but if you'd like to make your own, here are some recipes.

[GF] AMCHOOR (green mango powder)

Amchoor is also known as amchur, umchoor, aamchur, aampapad and amchor. It has a delicious sour, tangy, fruity flavor and a fragrance like honey. In India, this tangy condiment is made by slicing green (i.e. unripe) mangos, drying the slices in the sun and then grinding them to a powder. Amchoor is used in any dish where lemon could be used.

In India, both unripe and ripe mangos are used for making amchoor. The pulp from ripened mangos is sundried to make the sweet, golden-orange variety. Unripe mangos produce the sour and tangy amchoor that is considered a delicious gastronomic indulgence. In both cases the pulp is sun-dried, usually on a chattai (grass mat) in layers.

If you cannot obtain green mangos for tangy amchoor, you can make apple amchoor using tart cooking apples such as Granny Smith, or even under-ripe apples.[15] Studies suggest that compounds in unripe apples may even prevent the development of food allergies. [202]

---

14   Lavender oil has been shown to inhibit histamine release. [219]

15   Contrary to popular opinion, eating unripe apples does not necessarily make people sick. In fact, the United State Department of Agriculture states that the human stomach can digest both ripe and unripe apples. As long as you chew the apple sufficiently, it will not make you ill. Sufficient chewing, of course, aids in the digestive process.

The main difference between ripe and unripe apples is that unripe fruit contains substances which may cause gas to develop in the stomach, and this may cause problems for some people.

How to make amchoor

It is best to make only a small quantity at a time. Amchoor lasts a long time, even when used regularly, because it is strongly flavoured and only used sparingly.

It takes about 1 kilogram (2.2 pounds) of raw mangos to make about a cup of amchoor powder, which should last the average cook for a year!

> 1 kg (2.2 pounds) raw, unripe, green mangos

With a potato peeler, peel off the mango skins and discard the peels. Continuing to use the potato peeler, peel off strips of mango flesh and distribute them in a single layer in a sieve or a shallow basket. Discard the stones.

You can sun-dry the mango strips if the weather is hot enough, or use a food dehydrator or your oven to dry them.

To oven-dry:

Set your oven temperature as low as possible—this will probably be around 90° C (200° F). Space the cooking racks evenly apart if you are going to dry more than one tray of fruit.

Place a wire cooling rack on each of your baking trays. Spread the fruit out on the racks in one single, even layer. Place trays in the oven and turn on the fan, if fan-forced.

The drying process will take about 6 hours. During the drying, it may be necessary for you to turn the strips over occasionally, for faster, more even drying and to stop the strips from sticking together. Note: With fast drying, the mangos produce a lighter colored amchoor.

Dry the mango strips until they are completely desiccated and moisture-free. When they are ready, the strips will resemble potato crisps, and if you shake them they will rattle with a 'crisp' sound.

Place the dried mango strips in a food processor and process to a powder.

[GF] GREEN MANGO JUICE

The juice of unripe mangos is a boon to HIT sufferers. You don't realize how important to cooking are the zesty tang and acidic properties of vinegar and lemon juice, until you miss them. Fortunately the juice of green mangos makes a good substitute.

It's not widely available in stores, however; so if you cannot obtain it, you can substitute either amchoor (recipe below) or the juice of unripe/tart apples, mixed with a pinch of ascorbic acid powder.

To make your own green mango juice, buy unripe mangos and process them in a blender, then strain them through muslin to remove the pulp.

To store, freeze the juice in ice cube trays so that you can defrost as much as required in small amounts.

FRAGRANT, FLAVORED OILS

The safest method for making non-frozen oil infusions is to use herbs that have been dried, and people with HIT should avoid dried herbs if possible, so we will look at other methods.[16]

With the Strictly Low Histamine Diet, the freshness of food is crucial. However you might not always have access to fresh herbs and spices for flavoring—and flavor is especially important when one's diet is restricted. You may also want to make your own lemony herbs-infused oil as a good citrus-free, vinegar-free salad dressing. Freeze fresh herbs in oil and you will have them at hand at all times.

Some herbs have relatively hard leaves, which makes them suitable for simply chopping and freezing in oil. Rosemary,

---

16   Note: We recommend that you do not steep fresh herbs in oil in the home kitchen without freezing. 'The fresh vegetables, herbs, and/or fruits used to flavor or infuse oils can be contaminated with [Clostridium botulinum] spores. Fresh produce also contains water, which allows bacteria such as C. bot to live and grow. C. bot thrives in an oxygen-free environment like oil.' [211]

parsley, sage, oregano and other herbs with 'tough' leaves are best for freezing this way.

Softer-leafed herbs such as basil, mint, lemon verbena and dill are more delicate, and tend to lose their flavor when frozen by this method, so many cooks prefer to freeze them as a purée.

If you want to use the flavored oil without bits of leaf floating in it, simply strain the defrosted oil through a fine sieve or muslin cloth. Freezing bursts the plant cells, releasing the natural flavors and fragrances into the surrounding medium, so your home made herb oil will be full of flavor.

Flavored or infused oils can be used in dips, sauces, salads and marinades.

[GF] HARD-LEAFED HERB OILS

Using this method you can preserve herbs and make infused oils such as Rosemary Oil, Parsley Oil, Sage Oil, Lemon Myrtle Oil, Lemon Grass Oil, Coriander (cilantro) Oil, Oregano Oil etc.

> **your choice of fresh 'hard'-leafed herbs**
> **extra virgin olive oil, light olive oil, or rice bran oil**
> **ice cube trays**
> **plastic kitchen wrap**
> **freezer bags with ties**

Buy or pick your fresh herbs, wash them, dry them well on paper towel or in a salad dryer, then chop them and pack them tightly into the compartments of an ice cube tray. Do not mix different varieties of herbs.

Fill each compartment to the top with the oil of your choice. Light olive oil and rice bran oil have such a subtle flavor that they allow the taste of the herbs to really shine through.

Cover the tray lightly with plastic wrap and place it in the freezer for 24 hours.

Remove from the freezer, tip out the cubes and store them in an airtight freezer bag. Label each one with the name of the herb and the date. Replace in the freezer.

When herb-infused oil is required, defrost and strain the oil through a fine sieve or muslin.

[GF] HOME MADE ITALIAN SEASONING

> **3 tablespoons finely chopped basil**
> **3 tablespoons finely chopped oregano**
> **3 tablespoons finely chopped parsley**
> **1 tablespoon garlic powder**
> **1 teaspoon onion powder**
> **1 teaspoon finely chopped thyme**
> **1 teaspoon finely chopped rosemary**
> **½ teaspoon freshly cracked black pepper**

Mix all ingredients together, then freeze in oil to store, as explained in 'hard-leafed herb oils'.

[GF] SOFT-LEAFED HERB OILS

Using this method you can preserve herbs and make infused oils such as Basil Oil, Mint Oil, Peppermint Oil, Chocolate Mint Oil, Lemon Basil Oil, Lemon Balm Oil, Lemon Catmint Oil, Lemon Verbena Oil, Dill Oil, Red Shiso Oil, Green Shiso Oil and so on.

2 cups of fresh 'soft' herb leaves, lightly packed
½ cup of a low-odor vegetable oil such as light
**   olive oil, or rice bran oil**
a dash of green mango juice or amchoor
a pinch of salt
plastic zip-lock bags

You will end up with about ¼ the amount of purée, so for example if you begin with 4 cups of leaves you will get 1 cup of purée.

Wash the fresh herbs and pat them dry with paper towel or whizz them in a salad dryer. Pick the leaves off the stems and discard the stems.

Using either a mortar and pestle or a food processor, mash the leaves to a pulp and mix with the oil to form a purée. Add a few drops of green mango juice or a pinch of amchoor, and a pinch of salt.

Spoon the purée into plastic zip-lock bags, place the bags on a flat surface and pat them down gently so that the mixture spreads out thinly before you seal the bags. Label the bags and freeze them.

When herbs are needed for recipes, simply break off or cut off as much purée as required. When herb-infused oil is required, defrost and strain the oil through muslin.

[GF] SWEET FLAVORED OILS

Using the soft-leafed method to make sweet Rose Oil, Lemon Verbena Oil, Chocolate Mint Oil, Peppermint Oil, Cardamom Oil, Allspice Oil, Lavender Oil, Violet Oil or any sweet infused oil of your choice.

Omit the amchoor and salt and instead, add sugar—½ cup for every 2 cups of petals or leaves.

Before using sweet oil, defrost it and strain through muslin, pressing the petals or leaves to extract as much oil as you can.

[GF] FROZEN HERBS

If you do not have time to bother with oils, you can simply chop your herbs and place them in plastic bags, then press the bags out thinly, seal them and freeze them. The herbs will retain most of their color and fragrance, and you can break off the quantity you require.

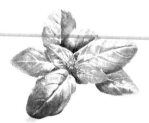

[GF] HIT-FRIENDLY DIJON MUSTARD

1 large onion, finely minced
3 cloves garlic, crushed
2 cups apple juice (from tart apples)
4 ounces dry wasabi powder
4 tablespoons honey
1 tablespoon mild oil (such as rice bran oil)
2 teaspoons salt

Combine the onion and garlic with the apple juice in a saucepan. Bring to a boil, then reduce the heat and simmer for 10 minutes.

Remove from heat and cool slightly. Pour through a strainer and discard the onion and garlic.

Add the dry wasabi powder to the flavored apple juice to make a paste. Add the honey, oil, and salt and mix well. Return the mixture to the saucepan and cook over a low heat until it thickens while you stir constantly. It will thicken by evaporation, so be patient.

Cool to room temperature, then mix well and store in a covered jar in the refrigerator.

Makes about 1 ½ cups

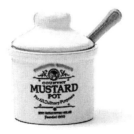

[GF] HIT-FRIENDLY MAYONNAISE

> 2 free-range egg yolks, at room temperature
> 2-3 teaspoons fresh green (unripe) mango juice[1]
> pinch of salt
> 100ml (3.5 fluid ounces) olive oil
> 100ml (3.5 fluid ounces) rice bran oil
> freshly ground white pepper
>
> ─────────
>
> 1   In emergencies you can substitute the juice of a
> very tart or unripe apple mixed with a pinch of ascorbic acid
> powder.

Place the egg yolks, 2 teaspoonsful of the green mango juice and the pinch of salt in the bowl of a food processor or blender and process until the mixture just begins to thicken.

Measure the olive and other vegetable oil into a jug. With the processor still running, slowly pour the oil into the egg-yolk mixture in a thin, steady stream, pausing sometimes to scrape down the inside of the blender with a spatula.

You must add the oil gradually, but not too slowly because the mixture could thicken too quickly. If this occurs add about 2 teaspoonsful of hot water to thin the mayonnaise before adding the rest of the oil.

Continue to blend until the mixture is thick, creamy and pale. Then taste the mayonnaise and adjust the seasoning with extra mango juice, salt and pepper if desired.

Transfer to a small, airtight container. Cover the surface of the mayonnaise with a piece of plastic wrap to prevent a skin from forming, then seal the container with the lid.

Store in the fridge and use within a few days. We do not recommend that you freeze it because it will separate.

NATURAL FOOD FLAVORINGS

COFFEE ESSENCES

Coffee essence is useful for baking, as well as for coloring and flavoring creams.

[GF] COFFEE ESSENCE—THE HOT METHOD

You can use instant coffee for this recipe, but for the best complexities of and depth flavor use espresso, percolated or plunger coffee made from your favorite coffee bean blend.

> **1 cup (8 fluid ounces) very strong, brewed coffee**
> **100 g (3 ½ ounces) sugar**

Place all ingredients in a small saucepan over a medium high heat and melt the sugar into the coffee while stirring.

Reduce the heat, then simmer the coffee for about 5 minutes. Remove from heat and allow to cool. Store in refrigerator.

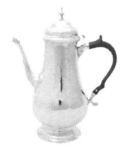

[GF] COFFEE ESSENCE—THE COLD METHOD

> **450 g (1 pound) ground coffee**
> **2.3 liters (10 cups) cold water**
> **2 x 3 liter jugs**
> **a coffee filter (or a large, plastic funnel lined with**
> **a cone of filter paper or muslin)**

Pour the coffee grounds into one of the jugs, then slowly fill the jug with cold water.

Allow the jug to stand undisturbed for at least 10 hours or overnight, but no more than 24 hours. Make sure you do not stir up or agitate the coffee grounds.

After the appropriate time has elapsed, set up the coffee filter over the other 3 liter jug. Carefully lift the full jug and pour the coffee gradually through the filter. When all the coffee has been filtered, allow the remaining grounds to sit in the filter and drain completely. This can take from several minutes to an hour.

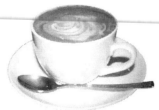

[GF] HERB AND FLOWER SUGARS

Using this method you can make sweet Rose Sugar, Lemon Verbena Sugar, Chocolate Mint Sugar, Peppermint Sugar, Cardamom Sugar, Allspice Sugar, Lavender Sugar, Violet Sugar or any sweet infused Sugar of your choice.

Basic Herb and Flower Sugars

Choose flowers that are free of pesticides. Roses, lavender or violets from a florist or nursery may not be chemical free.

Any roses will contain essential oils, but the Damask Rose (Rosa damascena) or the Cabbage Rose (Rosa centifolia) are the ones commercially cultivated for producing rose oil. Pick the roses in the morning, when their moisture and sugar levels are high. Gently wash the flowers to remove any insects or dirt.

Sweet Violets (Viola odorata) are a good source of vitamin C. They also contain rutin, a bioflavonoid which itself contains quercetin. Rutin has anti-inflammatory and antioxidant properties.

English Lavender (Lavandula angustifolia) is the only one to choose for making edible oils and sugars. Lavender is considered to be a natural antihistamine.

> **2 lightly packed measuring cups of fresh petals
>   or leaves**
> **½ cup to ¾ cup sugar**
> **plastic zip-lock bags**

Wash the fresh petals or leaves and pat them dry with paper towel or whizz them in a salad dryer. Pick them off the stems and discard the stems.

Place plant materials and sugar in a food processor and blend until they form a paste.

Spoon the paste into plastic zip-lock bags, place the bags on a flat surface and pat them down gently so that the mixture spreads out thinly before you seal the bags. Label the bags and freeze them.

Herb and flower sugars can be used to flavor drinks and desserts such as stewed fruit.

Lemon verbena sugar makes delicious lemon curd and lemon sponge cake. It has a lighter, more aromatic flavor than any of the other lemony herbs such as lemon balm or lemon grass.

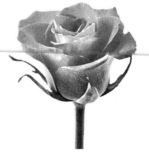

[GF] APPLE CARAMEL

> **1 liter (approx. 4 cups) of pure apple juice**

Pour apple juice into a large saucepan. Place pan over a high heat and bring it to the boil. Turn down the heat and simmer until the liquid decreases in quantity and turns a darker color. This could take between 30-60 minutes depending on the saucepan's size and how hot it gets.

After the first 10 minutes of simmering, make certain you check it frequently to ensure it does not scorch or burn.

To find out how thick it's getting, simply stir it with a wooden spoon. The longer it cooks, the thicker the apple caramel will become.

When you think it is ready, test it by scooping out a small spoonful, dropping it into a small, chilled bowl or saucer and waiting until it cools down. If it has 'syrupy' qualities, it's ready. If you want it thicker, cook a little longer.

Wearing protective oven mitts, carefully pour this very hot mixture gradually into a ceramic jar or bowl, cover with a lid and store in the refrigerator.

It may have hardened by the time you wish to use it, but if you leave it at room temperature for a while, or place the jar inside a bowl of boiling water, it will melt rapidly.

Use apple caramel as a natural food coloring and flavoring.

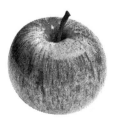

NATURAL FOOD COLORINGS

Some substances are both a coloring and a flavoring, as in the case of coffee essence {page 123} and caramel essence.

[GF] CARAMEL ESSENCE

This is both a natural food flavoring and a natural brown coloring

> **1 cup brown sugar, firmly packed**
> **2 tablespoons water**
> **1 cup boiling water**

Place sugar and 2 tablespoons water into a saucepan and set over a medium low heat. Cook, stirring continuously, until sugar is dissolved (about 2 minutes).

Slowly add 1 cup boiling water. Continue to cook the mixture for about 15 minutes, until it thickens and becomes syrupy.

This dark caramel syrup can be used to color stir-fry sauces.

[GF] PURPLE OR BLUE FOOD DYES

From Cabbage:

> **leaves of red or purple cabbage, sliced**
> **water**
> **baking powder**

Put the sliced cabbage leaves into a medium saucepan with enough water to cover them, and boil for 10-15 minutes.

Strain out the cabbage, return the colored water to the saucepan and bring to the boil again.

When boiling, turn the heat to low and simmer until the liquid has reduced to about a quarter of a cup (by evaporation).

After the liquid is reduced it will be thick and syrupy and intensely purple. This can be used as a food dye—the flavor is virtually imperceptible.

For a blue dye, add a tiny pinch of baking powder. If you add too much, you'll end up with a green food coloring that tastes fairly unpleasant. Keep adding baking soda in tiny amounts until the color just turns blue.

Use your purple or blue edible dye drop by drop, very sparingly, to add color to icings, cake batters and cookies.

Note: If you add the blue to an acidic food, it will turn back to purple and you'll have to add a little more baking soda.

Likewise if you add the purple to an alkaline food it will turn very strong blue and you'll have to add a pinch of something acidic, such as amchoor.

From Butterfly Pea:

You can buy dried butterfly pea flowers (*Clitoria ternatea*) online from websites such as Etsy.com and Alibaba.com. If you have a garden in the tropics, or a hothouse in temperate climates, you can grow your own, from seed.

To extract the vibrant blue color, steep 12 dried or fresh butterfly pea flowers in 1 cup boiling water for 15 minutes or until no color remains in the petals. Strain the blue liquid and discard the flowers. This is your food dye.

To obtain a purple or purplish-red color, add a tiny pinch of amchoor, which is acidic.

[GF] MAGENTA FOOD DYE

Magenta Plant (Peristrophe roxburghiana) is known in Vietnam as *lá cẩm*.

Wash a bunch of leaves and stalks well, and boil in 1 cup of water for 15 minutes. Squeeze gently to extract more color, then strain the liquid and discard residue.

[GF] RED FOOD DYES

Beetroots contain a brilliant red dye. Concentrated beet juice can be used as a red food coloring.

Pomegranate juice also makes a colorful food dye.

Rhubarb's red pigment leaches out during cooking. Save the cooking liquid, reduce it by simmering until most of it evaporates, leaving a thick syrup, and use this concentrated extract as a food coloring.

Hibiscus food coloring can be made the same way, and is a vivid, ruby red. Boil petals in water, then reduce the liquid. You can mix this infusion with sugar to make a colorful, flavorful hibiscus syrup. Dried hibiscus is widely available as a herbal tea.

[GF] YELLOW AND ORANGE FOOD DYES

Turmeric and saffron yield excellent and very stable yellow and orange food dyes.

To extract colour from raw carrots, whizz them in a blender with oil or water, then strain and discard the residue.

[GF] GREEN FOOD DYES

To make your own green dye cook mild-flavored green vegetables (such as collard, turnip greens, lettuce or even broccoli) for about a minute, then plunge them into ice water.

Drain and squeeze out the water, then place the greens in a blender with just enough water (or oil) to liquefy them, and process until smooth.

You will end up with a concentrated green paste.

If you decide to use oil, you'll find it carries the green color a little better. Strain the oil before using, and store it frozen in ice cubes. If you store it in the refrigerator, use within a few days.

Your green food coloring will have a flavor of its own, so if you prefer a subtle flavor use the vegetables suggested above, but if you want a stronger, aromatic flavor, choose parsley, mint, basil or roquette (arugula).

11. Breakfasts

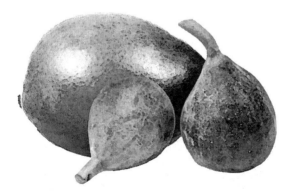

Breakfast can be a quick and easy meal. Oatmeal or oat bran porridge with added rice bran or wheat bran can help if you have a sluggish digestion. For a savory porridge add salt, as is traditional in Scotland. To make sweet porridge add stewed fruit and a sweetener of your choice. If you enjoy a creamier taste, stir in some mascarpone.

For a low carb breakfast, top a bed of roquette (aragula) leaves with scrambled egg yolks, and garnish with chopped chives or parsley.

Other breakfast choices include commercial rice or corn cereals with milk, gluten free waffles or pancakes, muesli, muffins, egg yolks cooked any style, toast (wheat-free) with jam (jelly), French toast, fresh fruit, fruit and vegetable smoothies, and egg yolks with fake bacon.

[GF] APPLE AND MANGO BIRCHER MUESLI

2 ½ cups rolled oats
1 ½ cups apple juice
1 cup cream ["Cream Substitutes" on page 106] or ricotta
¾ cup milk (low-fat or regular)
¾ cup or chopped sulfur-free dried mango
2 tablespoons honey or other sweetener [page 86]
¼ cup chopped, sulfur-free dried apple
3 fresh figs, quartered

Combine oats, apple juice, ricotta, milk, dried mango and honey in a medium bowl. Cover and refrigerate overnight, to allow oats and fruit to soften.

Next day, spoon muesli mixture into bowls. Sprinkle with dried apple. Top with fresh figs and serve.

[GF] WHEAT FREE SAVORY BREAKFAST MUFFINS

½ cup gluten free all-purpose plain flour
½ cup cornmeal or fine polenta
1 teaspoon baking powder
½ teaspoon baking soda
½ teaspoon salt
½ teaspoon pepper
½ cup parmesan substitute made with gluten free
    bread [page 110]
¼ cup fresh ricotta
2 tablespoons olive oil
2 free-range eggs
½ cup grated zucchini (courgette)
¼ cup chopped chives and parsley
¼ cup grated carrot
¼ cup sweet corn

Pre-heat oven to 180° C (350° F) and oil the cups of a muffin tray.

Beat together the polenta or cornmeal and flour, baking powder, baking soda, salt and pepper.

In a large bowl whisk together the ricotta, oil and egg yolks.

Add the flour mixture and remaining ingredients. Stir well until all ingredients are combined

With a spoon, dollop the mixture evenly into the muffin tray cups and bake for approximately 20 minutes.

Remove from oven and allow to cool in muffin tray for about 5 minutes before sliding a knife blade around the muffins to loosen them from the tray. Do not leave them cooling too long, or they might stick.

Turn them out and allow them to cool completely on a wire rack, or eat them warm.

These savory gluten free muffins are suitable to freeze. To serve, simply reheat in a microwave.

SMOOTHIES—DESIGN YOUR OWN

Smoothies retain all the beneficial fiber of the ingredients. They are a quick and flavorsome way to consume raw vegetables, particularly vegetables high in quercetin. Smoothies should consist of your chosen vegetable(s), a sweetener such as fresh fruit or any of the permitted sweeteners, some liquid and, if desired, a thickener such as apple purée or oat bran. To offset any bitterness from the greens, add a pinch of mango amchoor or a dash of green (unripe) mango juice.

[GF] GREEN GODDESS SMOOTHIE

2 handfuls permitted green leafy vegetables such
    as lettuce or bok choy
½ cup fresh basil
1 cup HIT-friendly milk of your choice
⅔ cup pieces of frozen mango or frozen
    cantaloupe (rock melon)
1 baby carrot
½ small cucumber
¼ cup raw broccoli florets
1 tablespoon freshly ground hemp seeds
a dash of amchoor or green mango juice
2 tablespoons cream

Combine all ingredients in a blender and process until very smooth, about 2 minutes. Pour into a glass and enjoy.

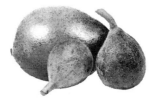

[GF] RED GODDESS SMOOTHIE

1 small beetroot, peeled
½ cup pomegranate juice
½ cup frozen stewed rhubarb
1 carrot
½ cup frozen watermelon pieces
1 cup unsweetened apple sauce/apple purée
½ cup honey or sweetener of your choice [page 86]
1 tablespoon oatmeal or oat bran (optional)

Combine all ingredients in a blender and process until very smooth, about 2 minutes. Pour into a glass and drink.

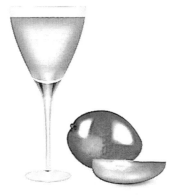

COMFORT-FOOD PORRIDGES

[GF] EASY HIGH FIBER OAT BRAN PORRIDGE

> **3 heaped tablespoons oat bran**
> **2 heaped tablespoons wheat bran**
> **¼ cup water**
> **oat milk, to serve**

Place the oat bran and wheat bran into a deep bowl. Add ¼ cup water and stir to mix. Microwave on 'high' for 1 ½ minutes. Serve with HIT-friendly milk of your choice.

[GF] SWEET OATMEAL PORRIDGE

> **3 cups milk or rice milk**
> **1 ½ cups traditional rolled oats**
> **pinch of salt**
> **1 ½ tablespoons brown sugar**
> **1 ripe mango, or 3 ripe figs, or ½ cup cantaloupe**
>   **(rock melon) sliced**
> **1 teaspoon ground cardamom**

Pour milk into a large saucepan and bring it to a simmer over medium-high heat. Add the oats and stir.

Bring the porridge to the boil, then reduce heat to medium.

Simmer, stirring with a wooden spoon, for 5 minutes or until porridge thickens (When it is thick enough it will coat the spoon). Take the saucepan off the heat, cover it with a lid and allow it to rest for 5 minutes to thicken a little more. Stir in salt and sugar.

Spoon into bowls. Top with fruit and cardamom. Serve.

Tip: instead of adding sugar you could drizzle the porridge with golden syrup, maple syrup or honey.

[GF] CELTIC OATMEAL PORRIDGE WITH HONEYED FIGS

Traditional Scottish and Irish porridge is made with steel-cut oats, not rolled oats. Steel-cut oats are made by slicing the whole oat groat (the inside of the oat kernel) with a steel blade. Sometimes they are called pinhead oats or Irish oats. Unlike rolled oats, steel-cut oats retain bits of the bran layer.

These golden grains are slower to cook than rolled oats, but have a delicious, nutty flavor and are lower on the glycaemic index.

> 1 cup steel-cut oats
> 4 cups water
> ½ teaspoon fine sea-salt
> 3 cups freshly made apple juice
> 2 fresh figs cut into quarters (or ⅓ cup stewed rhubarb)
> ¼ cup honey

Beat oats into 4 cups of rapidly boiling water, then reduce heat to a simmer. Cook for 30 minutes, stirring occasionally to prevent sticking.

While the oats are cooking, combine apple juice, honey and figs in a small pot over medium-low heat. Simmer uncovered, until most of the liquid has evaporated. There should be about 1 cup remaining—⅔ the original volume. Remove from heat and allow to cool a little.

When the oatmeal is cooked, stir in the salt. Spoon into bowls and top with fig mixture.

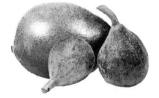

[GF] SAVORY OATMEAL PORRIDGE

¼ cup onion, finely chopped
1 cup vegetable stock ["[GF] Basic Vegetable
   Stock" on page 160]
½ cup rolled oats
½ cup fresh or frozen sweetcorn
½ teaspoon dried oregano or sage
¼ teaspoon cumin powder
1 tablespoon mango or apple amchoor [page
   114]
salt and pepper, to taste
butter, a walnut-sized knob (optional)
To garnish:
1 tablespoon cream of your choice [page 106]
¼ cup chopped parsley, coriander (cilantro) or
   chives

In a medium saucepan over a medium high heat, fry the onions in the stock until they become translucent.

Add the rest of the stock and turn up the heat.

When liquid begins to boil, add oats and corn. Return to the boil, then reduce heat to medium.

When ¾ of the liquid has been absorbed, stir in the cumin, oregano or sage, amchoor and salt and pepper.

Once the porridge has thickened to your desired consistency, serve it in a bowl with a dash of oat milk (or other milk of your choice).

Garnish with cream and fresh, chopped herbs.

[GF] BROWN RICE PORRIDGE

> 1 cup short-grain brown rice, cooked
> 1 tablespoon ground linseeds
> 1 cup HIT-friendly milk of your choice
> 1 teaspoon salt
> 2 drops natural oil-based vanilla essence
> 1 pinch cardamom powder
> sweetener of your choice [page 86] (optional)

Put rice and water in a pot, bring it to the boil and allow to simmer until the rice is cooked and the water is absorbed.

Add the milk and salt and gradually heat up the mixture, stirring frequently so that the milk does not stick and burn.

Simmer—do not boil—on a low heat for about 30 minutes, or until the porridge is thick.

Just before serving, stir in the natural caramel extract. Top with a sprinkling of spice and a drizzle of maple syrup or other sweetener.

About corn porridge

The difference between polenta and hominy: both hominy and polenta are made from stone-ground cornmeal. Most polenta is made from a class of corn called 'flint corn', a yellow corn that holds its coarse texture well.

Most hominy is made from a class of corn called 'dent corn', which has a very different texture and is usually pale in color. Hominy is made by simmering dent corn kernels in an alkaline solution of either lime ('pickling lime') or lye. This corrosive solution detaches the outer hull from the corn kernel and causes the grain to swell.

Cooked hominy is called 'grits', a surprising term given that the dish is soft and mushy, and not gritty at all—however the word 'grits' derives from the Old English word 'grytt', meaning coarse meal. This word originally referred to wheat and other cereals now known as 'groats' in parts of the UK.

[GF] POLENTA PORRIDGE

2 cups HIT-friendly milk of your choice
2 cups water
1 teaspoon coarse salt
1 cup polenta[1]
2 tablespoons rice bran oil (optional)

---

1   If polenta is unobtainable, substitute an equal amount of yellow cornmeal; but cook for only half the time.

Place the first 3 ingredients into a large, heavy saucepan and bring them to the boil over a medium-high heat.

Wearing a heatproof glove, take up a long-handled wooden spoon. Polenta can spit while cooking, and hot polenta can burn the skin.

While whisking the boiling water gently with the wooden spoon, pour the polenta into it in a steady stream.

Reduce heat to low, simmer until the polenta is smooth and thick, stirring almost constantly. The polenta will take about 18 minutes to thicken properly.

Just before serving, stir in the rice bran oil. Sprinkle polenta with salt and pepper for a savory porridge, or if you prefer, a sweetener. ["Sweeteners" on page 86]

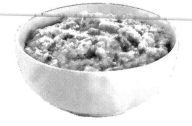

[GF] HOMINY GRITS

> **1 cup coarsely-ground hominy grits**
> **5 cups water or stock [page 160]**[1]
> **1 teaspoon salt**
> **2 tablespoons butter or vegetable oil (such as rice bran oil)**
>
> ———————
>
> 1   If you prefer a thicker consistency, use only 4 ½ cups of stock or water.

Put the stock or water into a large, heavy saucepan and bring it to a boil. Turn down the heat down to medium, and while the liquid is simmering, slowly beat in the grits, stirring continuously with a wooden spoon until they begin to thicken. This should take about 3-5 minutes.

Turn down the heat to low so that the mixture bubbles once or twice every few seconds, but is not at a rolling boil.

Simmer for 40-50 minutes. Coarse-ground grits will take longer to cook than fine-ground ones. Stir the mixture often so that the grits do not stick to the pan and burn.

You can tell when the grits are cooked through, because they become tender. When they are ready, whisk in the butter or oil and salt and serve steaming hot.

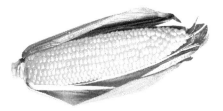

BREAKFAST EGGS

Nutritious, versatile, free-range egg yolks can be fried with HIT-friendly bacon ["HIT-friendly 'bacon'" on page 106], scrambled, boiled, poached, baked, steamed, made into omelets, slices, frittatas or quiches, or added to egg salads.

[GF] EASY SCRAMBLED EGGS

> **2 free-range egg yolks**
> **30 ml (1 fluid ounce) milk/cream of your choice [page 106]**
> **a splash of rice bran oil for frying**
> **toasted gluten-free bread ["16. Breads" on page 193], buttered, to serve**
> **chopped herbs, to garnish (parsley, chives etc.)**

Beat egg yolks and cream together in a bowl until combined. Season with salt and pepper.

Melt butter in a saucepan over medium heat. Pour egg mixture into pan. Stir continuously while egg mixture is cooking, so that all cooks evenly.

When the mixture has set into tender, fluffy curds (about 2 minutes) immediately remove pan from heat. Note: Overcooking causes the mixture to separate and become watery.

Serve egg yolks on toast, sprinkled with chopped herbs and accompanied by a side dish of steamed asparagus tips.

BREAKFAST 'HAMMAN EGG' PIES

We can't call these 'ham and egg' pies because they don't contain any ham. But they taste great.

80g bacon substitute [page 106]
4 egg yolks, at room temperature
1 teaspoon sumac, amchoor [page 114] or
   ascorbic acid powder
2 tablespoons flat-leaf parsley leaves, chopped
1 tablespoon ricotta cheese or rice cream
   [page 106]
1 tablespoon HIT-friendly thickened cream of
   your choice
30g roquette (aragula) leaves, trimmed
salt and black pepper, according to your taste
4 slices crusty bread [page 193], toasted, to serve

Preheat oven to 180°C. Grease four ½-cup capacity ovenproof ramekins and line the base and sides with 'bacon bits'.

Crack 1 egg into each ramekin. Top each egg with a quarter of the sumac (or amchoor), parsley and crumbled ricotta or rice cream. Drizzle 1 teaspoon of thickened cream over each. Season with salt and pepper.

Bake pies in the oven for 15 to 18 minutes for soft yolks, or until egg is cooked to your preference. Remove from the oven and allow them to rest for 2 to 3 minutes.

Divide roquette (aragula) leaves between plates. Turn out hamman egg pies and place on top of leaves. Serve with toast.

BREAKFAST OMELET

> **2 free-range egg yolks**
> **1 tablespoon cold water (for a lighter, fluffier omelet)**
> **salt and ground white pepper**
> **15g (½ ounce) butter or HIT-friendly butter substitute**
> **buttered toast, to serve [page 193]**

Crack the eggs into a jug and separate the yolks from the whites. Discard the whites. Add the water to the yolks and beat with a fork until well mixed, then season with salt and pepper.

Put the butter in a medium-sized frypan over medium-high heat and melt it until it begins to bubble, but do not allow it to burn. Pour in the egg mixture, tilting the pan slightly to cover the base.

As the omelet cooks, use a spatula to gently draw the outer edges of the omelet towards the center, so that any uncooked egg runs underneath to cook.

Fry for 1-2 minutes or until the base of the omelet is set and a pale golden color, and the top is still slightly moist. This moist top will continue to cook and set more firmly after the omelet is folded over for serving. A tender omelet tastes far better than a dry, over-cooked one.

Slide a spatula under the edge of the omelet that is closest to you, and fold it towards the middle. Next, fold over the other edge.

Tilt the pan away from you and briskly flip the omelet onto a warmed serving plate. Serve straight away, with hot buttered toast.

[GF] BREAKFAST FRITTATA

rice bran oil spray
1 tablespoon rice bran oil
500g (one pound) fresh mixed vegetables
    such as broccoli, cauliflower, zucchini
    (courgette), green beans, cabbage, sweet
    corn, leeks, Chinese cabbage, spring
    onions (scallions), celery, snap peas,
    asparagus, carrot, parsnip etc.
6 free-range egg yolks
125ml (½ cup) milk
salt and pepper
freshly torn salad leaves, to serve

Preheat oven to 180°C (350°F). Prepare a square cake pan with a base measurement of 20cm (8 inches), by spraying it with rice bran oil. Line the base and sides with non-stick baking paper (parchment paper), allowing the two long sides to overhang.

Chop the vegetables into bite sized pieces.

Next, pour the oil into a large non-stick frying pan and place it over a medium-high heat.

Stir-fry the freshly chopped vegetables for 3 minutes or until soft. Pour them into the prepared cake pan.

Whisk egg yolks and milk in a bowl until thoroughly mixed. Season with salt and pepper according to your taste, and pour the mixture over the vegetables.

Place inside the oven and bake for 25-30 minutes or until set, firm and light golden in color.

Remove frittata from the oven and allow to stand for 10 minutes to cool slightly.

Serve with a crisp, green salad.

[GF] FLUFFY GLUTEN-FREE PANCAKES

**125g (½ cup) gluten free all-purpose plain flour
    with permitted ingredients
1 free-range egg
250ml (1 cup) oat milk [page 94]
a knob of butter, for frying**

Pour the flour into a mixing bowl and make a 'well' in the center.

Break the egg into the well and add a quarter of the milk. Whisk thoroughly to combine the mixture.

When the mixture forms a paste, add another quarter cup of milk and continue to whisk out any lumps. When the mixture is smooth, pour in the last of the milk.

Allow the mixture to stand for 20 minutes, then stir it again.

Place butter in a small, non-stick frypan on a medium heat. When the butter starts to bubble, pour a small quantity of the pancake batter into the pan and swirl around to coat the base with a thin layer.

Fry on a medium heat (so that the butter does not burn) for a few minutes until the pancake is golden brown on the bottom, then flip it over and fry until toasty brown on the other side.

Repeat the process until all the batter has been used, stirring the batter between pancakes and adding more butter for frying as necessary.

Serve with honey and a sprinkling of amchoor, or top with cream and stewed apple or figs, or sliced mango and maple syrup.

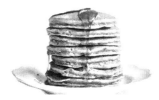

[GF] MESOPOTAMIAN HEMPSEED PANCAKES

1 ⅓ cups hempseed meal
⅔ cup water-chestnut flour
3 teaspoons baking powder
½ teaspoon salt (or to taste)
1 ½ tablespoons olive oil
4 free-range egg yolks
rice bran oil spray
unsweetened applesauce (approx. 2 tablespoons)
a knob of HIT-friendly butter, for frying

In a bowl, thoroughly mix together the dry ingredients. In a separate smaller bowl, lightly whisk the egg yolks. Pour eggs into dry ingredients.

Add applesauce gradually, mixing well, until the batter reaches your desired texture. Make the batter thin enough to spread on a hot cast iron frypan.

Place butter in a small, non-stick frypan on a medium heat. When the butter starts to bubble, pour a small quantity of the pancake batter into the pan and swirl around to coat the base with a thin layer.

Fry on a medium heat (so that the butter does not burn) for a few minutes until the pancake is golden brown on the bottom, then flip it over and fry until toasty brown on the the other side.

Repeat the process until all the batter has been used, stirring the batter between pancakes and adding more butter for frying as necessary.

Serve hot in a stack.

Topping: Amchoor or sumac sprinkled over a drizzle of maple syrup or honey.

[GF] SWEET POTATO HASH BROWNS WITH APPLE AND ONION MARMALADE

2 sweet potatoes
¼ cup white onion, finely chopped
4 garlic cloves, minced
¼ cup permitted gluten free flour (oat, brown
    rice, millet etc.)
1 teaspoon salt
½ teaspoon freshly ground black pepper
rice bran oil for frying

Wash and peel sweet potatoes, then grate (shred) them. Place the shredded sweet potato in a colander and rinse under cold water until the water runs mostly clear. (When you cut a tuberous vegetable, a small quantity of starch remains on the cut surface. Then when you fry it, the starch may brown at a more rapid rate than the inside of the potato cooks; consequently your hash browns may end up undercooked. Rinsing removes starch fro the surface.)

Squeeze the rinsed sweet potatoes to remove excess liquid, and put them into a medium sized bowl.

Add flour, garlic, onion, salt and pepper, and mix until all are thoroughly combined.

Add 2 tablespoons of frying oil to a cast iron or standard frypan and place over a medium-high heat.

Test the pan by throwing in a few sweet potato shreds. If they crackle, the pan is hot enough.

Use a ¼ cup to measure the grated sweet potato into the pan and then flatten out each hash brown with the back of a spatula.

Fry for about 3 minutes until crisp and golden-brown, then turn over the hash browns and fry for about 2 more. Cooking times vary, according to the heaviness of our frypan and your stove's individual heat settings.

As the hash browns finish cooking, remove them from the frypan, slide them onto a plate lined with paper towel and let them drain and cool for a short while.

Serve topped with onion marmalade or poached egg. Makes: 12 hash browns.

Apple and Onion Marmalade

1 tablespoon rice bran oil
1 teaspoon wasabi powder
2 large onions, diced
½ cup apple juice
½ cup chicken stock or vegetable stock ["HIT-friendly Chicken Stock" on page 161]
2 cooking apples[1], peeled, cored and diced into 1.5 cm (½-inch) pieces
¼ teaspoon salt
¼ teaspoon freshly ground black pepper
⅛ teaspoon ground allspice
2 tablespoons chopped fresh flat-leaf (Italian) parsley

---

1   We recommend Granny Smith apples, because of their sharp acidity and the fact that they hold their shape well when cooked.

Put the rice bran oil into a straight-sided frypan and place it over a medium heat. Add the wasabi and onions and cook, stirring occasionally, for about 10 minutes or until the onions become pale golden.

Pour in the apple juice and stock and bring to a boil over high heat. Add the apples, pepper, salt and allspice.

Turn down the heat to low and simmer, uncovered, about 12 minutes or until the apples are tender.

Take the frypan off the heat and mix in the chopped parsley.

Serve the marmalade warm or at room temperature.

Apple and onion marmalade keeps for up to a week in the refrigerator, if kept in a container with a tight-fitting lid, but make sure you warm it up before serving.

Makes about 2 cups.

FRENCH TOAST

> 4 large free-range egg yolks
> 1 teaspoon sugar (optional)
> pinch of salt
> 1 cup rice milk, oat milk or HIT-friendly milk of
>   your choice
> 10 to 12 slices white bread ["Breads" on page 193]
> butter or HIT-friendly butter substitute
> maple syrup or other syrup

Place egg yolks into a wide, shallow bowl or pie plate. Whisk lightly with a fork. Mix in sugar, salt, and milk.

Put a knob of butter into a frypan, and place the frypan over a medium-low heat. Melt the butter, tipping the frypan back and forth until it forms a thin layer.

Put the bread slices, one at a time, into the egg and milk mixture. Allow each slice to soak for a few seconds before gently flipping it to coat the other side. Soak only as many slices as you can fit in the frypan in one batch.

Transfer the soaked bread slices to the frypan and cook slowly until the undersides turn golden brown. Flip the slices over and brown the other side.

Serve French toast hot with butter and syrup.

Serves 4 people.

BAKED EGGS WITH HERBS

8 free-range egg yolks
160ml (½ cup) thick, whipped HIT-friendly
    cream of your choice
2 green shallots or spring onions, thinly sliced
¼ cup finely chopped fresh chives
salt and freshly ground black pepper
rice bran oil
toasted bread ["16. Breads" on page 193], sliced
    into fingers, to serve
HIT-friendly butter for the toast

Preheat oven to 200°C. Brush the insides of eight 125ml (½-cup) capacity ovenproof ramekins with rice bran oil.

Break an egg into each ramekin.

Pour the cream onto the egg yolks, sharing it evenly among ramekins. Sprinkle the chopped vegetables over the top and season with salt and pepper.

Set ramekins on a baking tray in the oven, and cook for 10 minutes or until egg yolks are set according to your preference.

Serve hot, accompanied by buttered toast fingers.

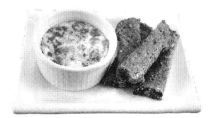

12. Entrées and Soups

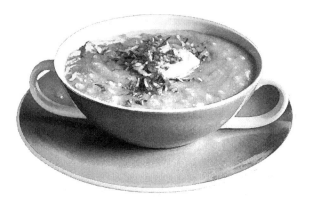

[GF] PINK PARTY DIP

> **650g (about 3) fresh, young beetroots, trimmed**
> **80ml (⅓ cup) rice bran oil**
> **2 cloves garlic, crushed**
> **280g (1 cup) oat cream, cornstarch cream or ricotta**
> **salt to taste**

Preheat oven to 180°C (350°F). Put beetroots in a bowl with 2 tablespoons oil and shake them until they are coated with the oil. Add salt and pepper according to your taste.

Wrap each beetroot loosely in foil, put them in a shallow, ovenproof dish and roast for an hour and a half, or until they are tender (use a skewer to test). Unwrap them and allow them to cool to room temperature.

Grate the beetroots coarsely, then leave them in a colander to drain off excess juice. Mix together the beetroots, the remaining 2 tablespoons. oil, the garlic and the cream in a large bowl, then sprinkle with a pinch of salt and pepper. Yields two cups of dip.

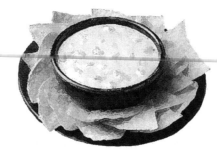

CRUSTY ITALIAN CROSTINI

> **1 stick or loaf of bread ["Breads" on page 193]**
> **cut into 1cm (½ inch) thick slices**
> **½ cup olive oil or rice bran oil**
> **2 teaspoons freshly ground coriander (cilantro)**
> **seeds**
> **2 teaspoons freshly ground black cumin**
> **1 teaspoon onion powder**
> **salt and pepper to taste**

Preheat oven to 200°C (400°F). Lay the bread slices, in a single layer, on two large baking trays.

In a bowl, mix together the oil, coriander (cilantro), cumin, onion powder, salt and pepper. Brush both sides of each slice with oil mixture.

Bake the slices for 10 minutes. Use oven tongs to turn them over and bake for another 10 minutes or until golden and crisp. Set aside to cool before serving.

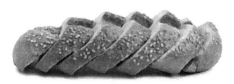

FRENCH ONION SOUP WITH GARLIC BREAD

Soup:

60g butter or HIT-friendly butter substitute,
    chopped
2 tablespoons olive oil
6 medium-large brown onions, thinly sliced
2 teaspoons brown sugar
2 tablespoons plain flour with permitted ingredients
4 cups vegetable stock [1] [page 160]

---

1   Do not use commercial stock cubes.

Garlic bread:

12 bread slices ["16. Breads" on page 193], each
    1.5cm thick (or any yeast-free seed-free, wheat-
    free bread with allowed ingredients)
olive oil cooking spray
1 tablespoon crushed garlic
1 cup softened butter
1 tablespoon salt, and pepper to taste

To make soup: In a saucepan with a heavy base, heat butter and oil over a medium-low heat until they are sizzling. Stir in the sliced onions and 1 teaspoon salt. Cook the mixture, uncovered, stirring frequently, for about 45 minutes or until the onions are very soft. Combine the sugar with the onions and cook, stirring frequently, for 10 more minutes or until the onions caramelize.

Next add the flour to the saucepan and continue to cook and stir the mixtire for two minutes.

Pour in the stock and 2 cups water. Turn down the heat to 'low' and simmer the soup, uncovered, for 15 minutes to permit the flavours to mingle.

To make garlic bread: Preheat oven to 180°C.

Beat the crushed garlic into the butter, then spread it on both sides of each slice of bread. Arrange the slices on 2 baking trays. Bake, turning once at the halfway point, for 10 to 12 minutes or until bread is light golden.

Ladle the hot soup into bowls. Top each serving with garlic bread, season with pepper and serve.

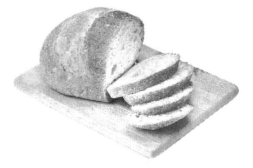

CREAMY INDIVIDUAL SOUFFLÉS

> 1 tablespoon HIT-friendly butter, to grease ramekins
> ⅓ cup ricotta
> 1 teaspoon prepared wasabi
> 1 teaspoon oregano
> pinch of pepper
> ¼ cup finely chopped chives
> 85g HIT-friendly Parmesan cheese [page 110]
> 3 tablespoons oat milk or milk of your choice
> 3 free-range egg yolks, separated
> salt, to taste

Preheat oven to 200° C (400° F)

Lavishly butter 6 ceramic ramekins, each one able to hold approximately ½ cup.

Place the ricotta, the wasabi, oregano, pepper, chives, HIT-friendly Parmesan, oat milk and 3 egg yolks in a bowl and beat them until well mixed.

Pour the egg whites into a small, deep bowl (preferably copper, stainless-steel, or glass) with a rounded bottom, and add the salt. Both your bowl and beaters must be completely clean and dry, or your egg whites won't whip properly.

Using a whisk or beaters, whip the salted egg whites until stiff peaks form. Test by lifting the beaters straight up from the egg whites. Snowy peaks should form and stand on top of the mixture, and when you tilt the bowl, the egg whites should not slide about.

Be careful not to overbeat, or the whites will become dry and clump together.

Immediately fold the stiff egg whites into the milky batter. Work rapidly so that the egg whites don't have time to collapse. Scoop some batter into each ramekin. Place ramekins into a baking pan or bain marie filled with enough hot water to come three-quarters of the way up their sides.

Place the pan in the pre-heated oven and bake for about 15 minutes. The soufflés will rise a little, but not to a very great height. When they are cooked, they should still be soft in the middle.

Leave them inside their ramekins to serve.

Makes 6 soufflés.

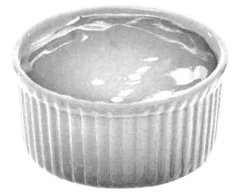

[GF] BASIC VEGETABLE STOCK

1 tablespoon olive oil
2 large brown onions, coarsely chopped
1 medium sized swede (rutabaga), peeled,
    coarsely chopped
2 carrots, peeled, coarsely chopped
4 celery sticks, coarsely chopped
3 liters/12 cups (100 fluid ounces) cold water
6 fresh parsley stalks
10 whole black peppercorns
3 dried bay leaves

Heat the oil in a large stockpot over medium-high heat. Add the onion, swede (rutabaga), carrot and celery and cook, stirring, for 5 minutes or until vegetables are brown.

Add the water, parsley, peppercorns and bay leaves, turn up the heat and bring the mixture to the boil. Use a metal sieve or a fine-slotted spoon to remove any scum that floats to the surface.

Reduce heat to medium-low and simmer, uncovered, for 2 hours, skimming the surface every 30 minutes.

Remove from heat. Set aside for 30 minutes to cool slightly.

Place a fine sieve over a large heatproof bowl. Carefully strain stock through the sieve.

Discard the solids from the sieve (they make excellent compost for your garden). Cool the stock to room temperature.

Note: You can either store the stock in the refrigerator in an airtight container, or freeze it in ice cubes, then pop out the ice cubes, seal them in freezer bags and store them in the freezer. Each time you cook, you only need to defrost as much as required.

[GF] HIT-FRIENDLY CHICKEN STOCK

> **2 cups dry brown, black, red or purple rice,
>   soaked overnight**
> **6 cups celery, chopped**
> **3 cups carrots, chopped**
> **2 cups onions, chopped**
> **4 cups orange-fleshed sweet potato, chopped**
> **1 cup potato, chopped**
> **2 cups apple, chopped**
> **½ cup garlic, chopped**
> **1 teaspoon fresh turmeric, chopped (or ¼ tea-
>   spoon ground)**
> **5 bay leaves**
> **1 ¼ cup parsley, chopped**
> **2 ½ tablespoon fresh oregano, chopped**
> **2 tablespoons fresh sage, chopped**
> **4 ½ tablespoons fresh rosemary, chopped**
> **1 tablespoon peppercorns**
> **½ teaspoon salt**
> **470 ml (5 quarts) water**

Place all the ingredients into a large stock pot and stir to combine. Bring the mixture to a boil, then the reduce heat, cover with a lid and simmer it for about an hour.

Strain the broth through a colander into a large bowl. With a wooden spoon, stir and push the contents of the colander to squeeze out as much liquid as possible, then discard the solids.

Wash out the stock pot, then strain the broth back into it to extract as much solid matter as you can. Finally, pour it through a fine strainer layered with cheesecloth, to achieve a clear, flavorsome broth. Fresh herbs will give a clearer broth than dried herbs or powders. You should end up with about 4 quarts of flavorsome broth, which can be added to casseroles, stews and soups.

ITALIAN VEGETABLE SOUP

1 tablespoon olive oil
1 large zucchini (courgette), finely chopped
1 medium fennel bulb, finely chopped
1 large carrot, peeled and finely chopped
2 garlic cloves, crushed
150 ml (⅓ pint) HIT-friendly chicken stock
    substitute
75g (⅓ cup) cooked brown rice
85g (½ cup) fresh green peas
1 tablespoon finely chopped fresh tarragon
salt and pepper
sliced toast, to serve ["16. Breads" on page 193]

Put the oil into a large saucepan and place it over a high heat. When it is hot, add the garlic, carrot, fennel and zucchini and cook, stirring frequently, for 5 minutes or until just tender.

Pour in the HIT-friendly chicken stock and bring the soup to the boil. Add the rice and peas and cook for 2 minutes or until peas are tender, but have not lost their color.

Remove from heat and stir in the tarragon, salt and pepper. Serve the soup steaming hot, with toast.

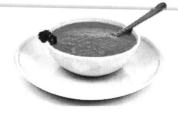

[GF] BROCCOLI AND SWEET POTATO SOUP

> 1 tablespoon olive oil
> 1 large brown onion, chopped
> 1kg (2 pounds) broccoli florets
> 2 sweet potatoes, peeled and chopped
> 2 garlic cloves, crushed
> 2 cups vegetable stock ["[GF] Basic Vegetable
>   Stock" on page 160]

Heat oil in a large saucepan over medium-high heat. Add onion and garlic. Cook, stirring, for 3 minutes or until the vegetables are soft.

Add broccoli, sweet potato, vegetable stock and 2 cups cold water. Cover with a lid and bring to the boil.

Reduce heat to low and simmer the soup, stirring occasionally, for 10 to 15 minutes or until sweet potato is tender.

Remove soup from heat and pour into a blender or use a hand-held stick blender to process until smooth.

Return soup to pan and cook for 5 more minutes or until heated through. Sprinkle with pepper before serving.

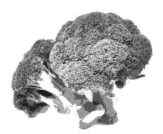

ZUCCHINI (COURGETTE) & DILL FRITTERS

600g zucchini (courgette), coarsely chopped
4 shallots, finely sliced
1 onion, grated
1 garlic clove, crushed
2 free-range egg yolks
150g (5 ounces) ricotta
1 tablespoon salt
½ teaspoon salt
½ teaspoon amchoor [page 114]
3 tablespoons parmesan substitute
3 tablespoons chopped fresh dill
3 slices bread ["16. Breads" on page 193], crusts
    removed
50g plain flour with permitted ingredients
4 tablespoons light olive oil
salad leaves, chopped cucumber, grated carrot/
    beetroot mix, and extra dill, to serve

Put the chopped zucchini in a colander, sprinkle with 1 table-spoon salt and set aside to drain for 30 minutes.

Meanwhile, thoroughly mix the ricotta with the ½ teaspoon salt and the amchoor.

Rinse the drained zucchini pieces under cold water, then wrap them in a clean tea towel and squeeze out excess moisture.

Place in a bowl mix in add shallots, onion, garlic, egg yolks, seasoned ricotta, HIT-friendly Parmesan and dill.

Taste the mixture and if you wish, season with salt and pepper.

Whiz the bread in a food processor until it turns into crumbs. Add the crumbs to the zucchini mixture and combine thoroughly. The mixture should now be quite dry—if not, throw in some extra crumbs.

Roll heaped tablespoons of the mixture into 12 balls, then flatten the balls slightly. Place flour in a bowl and roll the balls in the flour to coat them all over.

Heat oil in a non-stick frying pan, add fritters and cook in batches over medium heat for 1-2 minutes each side.

Layer salad leaves between fritters and serve with a topping of chopped cucumber, grated carrot and beetroot mix, and a garnish of dill.

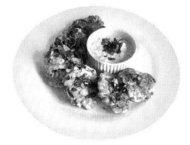

[GF] ZUCCHINI (COURGETTE) & SWEETCORN FRITTERS

> **310g (11 ounces) fresh or frozen sweetcorn kernels**
> **150g (5 ounces) zucchini, grated**
> **2 free-range egg yolks, lightly beaten**
> **⅓ cup oat milk, or other HIT-friendly milk of**
>   **your choice [page 94]**
> **1 cup gluten free self-raising flour with permitted**
>   **ingredients, sifted**
> **½ teaspoon ground black cumin seeds**
> **salt and pepper**
> **HIT-friendly sour cream, to serve**
> **coriander (cilantro) leaves, to garnish**

Beat together the milk, egg yolks, zucchini and sweetcorn. Slowly add the flour and black cumin, salt and pepper, while stirring continuously.

Place a 1 ½ tablespoons of rice bran oil in a non-stick frying pan over medium heat. When the oil is hot, place heaped table-spoonsful of the batter into the frypan and fry in batches until tiny bubbles begin to form on top.

Slide a spatula under each fritter check to see whether the underneath is golden brown. If it is, flip the fritter once, then continue to cook until golden brown on the other side and cooked through.

Drain off any excess oil on paper towel, cover the fritters and keep them warm until the whole batch is cooked.

Serve with a generous dollop of HIT-friendly sour cream [page 105], and garnish with coriander (cilantro).

Serves 4.

[GF] BLACK RICE FRITTERS WITH ARACAR SAUCE

For the Aracar sauce:
  ½ cup extra-virgin olive oil
  2 garlic cloves, peeled and crushed
  1 cup parsley leaves, lightly packed
  1 cup coriander (cilantro) leaves, lightly packed
  1 teaspoon salt
  ¼ teaspoon freshly ground black pepper
  1 tablespoon amchoor
  ¼ cup red onion, finely chopped.

Place the olive oil and garlic into a food processor or a mortar, and blend until well-mixed.

Add the parsley, coriander (cilantro), salt, pepper and amchoor, and blend until everything is mixed. Be careful not to overprocess and turn it to smooth mush; leave some texture.

Pour into a mixing bowl and stir in the onions.

Taste and modify salt, pepper and amchoor as needed.

For the black rice fritters:
  3 cups cooked and cooled black rice
  2 free-range egg yolks
  ½ teaspoon turmeric
  ½ teaspoon sumac
  ½ teaspoon salt
  ½ teaspoon black pepper
  1 tablespoon rice bran oil
  fine-ground rock salt

Place the egg yolks into a medium sized bowl and beat them lightly with a fork. Add the rice, turmeric, sumac, salt and pepper.

Cover a plate with paper towels. Swirl a tablespoon of rice bran oil in a large, heavy frypan over a medium high heat, to coat the pan.

Scoop ¼ cup of the rice mixture into the frypan and flatten it with the back of a spatula. Cook until golden brown underneath (this takes about 2 minutes, then turn it over and fry cook until the other side is golden brown.

Take the cooked fritters out of the frypan and allow them to drain on the paper towel-lined plate. Sprinkle with a pinch of fine rock salt.

Repeat the process until all the batter is used up. Serve steaming hot with Aracar sauce on the side, and a bowl of garden salad.

Serves 4

Note: Black rice requires longer cooking time than white rice. Soak and rinse it well, then cook with two cups of water to every one cup of rice. Usually the rice will need to cook for 25-30 minutes if it has been soaked or around one hour if un-soaked.

13. Main Courses

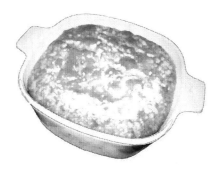

GARDEN FRITTATA

rice bran oil spray
200g (7 ounces) sweet potato, peeled, cut into 1cm
    (½ inch) pieces, rinsed in cold water and dried
120g (4 ounces) green beans, trimmed and halved
80g (3 ounces) frozen green peas
1 shallot, thinly sliced
125ml (4 fluid ounces) oat milk or other milk
    [page 94]
4 free-range egg yolks, lightly whisked
60g (2 ounces) HIT-friendly cream (low fat if you
    wish)
35g (1 ounce) HIT-friendly Parmesan [page 110]

Set your grill on medium-high to preheat. Take a non-stick, deep-sided over-proof frypan with a base measurement of 20cm (8 inches) and spray it with oil.

Place the frypan over a medium heat. and add sweet potato. Stir it while it cooks until slightly tender. This should take 3-4 minutes.

Add green beans. Continue to cook and stir for 1 minute, then add peas and cook for another minute or until beans and peas are soft but still crunchy.

Mix in the shallots and sprinkle with salt and pepper.

Beat milk, egg and cream in a jug and pour it over the cooked vegetables in the frypan. Tilt the pan to distribute the egg mixture evenly.

Reduce heat to medium-low and simmer for 8 minutes or until the frittata has almost set.

Sprinkle with HIT-friendly Parmesan and set the frypan under the grill. Grill for 3-5 minutes or until golden-brown on top.

Serves 4

[GF] BLACK RICE PILAF

⅓ cup rolled oats, toasted
1 ½ tablespoons rice bran oil
1 large brown onion, finely chopped
400g (14 ounces) frozen chopped mixed
    vegetables such as carrot, broccoli, cauliflower,
    peas and green beans
1 ½ cups black rice
1 teaspoon ground black cumin
1 teaspoon pepper
1 teaspoon allspice
1 teaspoon cardamom
¾ cup roughly chopped fresh coriander (cilantro)
    leaves

Heat oil in a large saucepan over medium heat. Add onion. Cook, stirring, for 3 minutes or until softened.

Add vegetables, rice and spices. Cook while stirring for 1 minute or until fragrant.

Mix in 2 cups cold water. Bring to the boil. Reduce heat to low. Cook, covered, for 15 minutes or until rice is tender and water has been absorbed.

Add half the toasted rolled oats and coriander (cilantro). Mix well.

Spoon into bowls. Serve garnished with remaining oats and coriander.

Serves 4

[GF] ASIAN STIR-FRY

Vegetables
1 onion, thinly sliced
100g (3.5 ounces) carrots, cut into matchsticks
225g (8 ounces) zucchini (courgette), sliced
175g (6 ounces) baby corn
225g (8 ounces) green beans, trimmed
½ stick celery, thinly sliced
250g (9 ounces) green or white cabbage
a pinch of amchoor [page 114] or sumac
4 tablespoons rice bran oil

Stir-fry sauce
1 teaspoon cornflour
2 tablespoons cold water
2 garlic cloves, crushed
50g (2 ounces) grated ginger
¼ teaspoon black pepper
¼ teaspoon salt
170ml (8 fluid ounces) olive oil or rice bran oil
2 teaspoons onion powder
½ teaspoon ground allspice
2 fresh or frozen kaffir lime leaves, stems
    discarded, cut into strips with scissors
1 tablespoon natural caramel coloring [page 128]
    or dark colored honey

To make the sauce, place cornflour and cold water in a small bowl and mix until they form a paste. Place all other sauce ingredients in a food processor and blend well to form a thick paste. Add the cornflour paste and blend thoroughly.

Taste-test the sauce for sweet and sour balance, adding more caramel if necessary. Set aside.

To cook the vegetables, pour oil into a wok and place over high heat. When oil is hot, add onion and cook for about 30 seconds. Add carrot, celery, zucchini and corn, and stir-fry for 1 minute. Add cabbage and continue cooking for about 30 seconds until cabbage becomes tender but is still crisp.

Stir in sauce and cook for long enough to just heat the sauce through.

[GF] PASTA WITH GARLIC AND BROCCOLI

> **500g (18 ounces) dry, gluten-free spaghetti pasta**
> **750g (26 ounces) broccoli, trimmed, cut into**
>   **small florets, stalks discarded**
> **2 garlic cloves, crushed**
> **⅓ cup olive oil**

Place pasta in a large saucepan of boiling, salted water, and cook until tender.

Add broccoli to the saucepan for the last 5 minutes of cooking. Pour pasta and broccoli into a colander and allow it to drain.

Pour oil into empty saucepan and return it to medium-high heat. Add garlic and cook, stirring, until fragrant. Return pasta and broccoli to pan, mix well and serve.

Serves 4

SWEET POTATO BASKETS

2 short, fat sweet potatoes, unpeeled, weighing
about 400g (14 ounces) each.
rice bran oil spray
2 teaspoons olive oil
1 teaspoons ground black cumin seeds
1 teaspoon onion powder
½ cup broccoli cut into small florets
1 small carrot, grated
2 tablespoons HIT-friendly cream (low fat if you
wish)
2 tablespoons HIT-friendly Parmesan [page 110]

Use a soft brush to scrub the sweet potatoes clean in cold water. Preheat oven to 180°C and line a baking tray with non-stick baking paper (parchment paper).

Slice the sweet potatoes in half crossways (as distinct from lengthways). Put them, cut side down, on the lined tray and spray them with oil.

Place in the oven and bake for 1 hour or until the flesh is soft and can easily be penetrated with a fork. Remove from oven and set aside for 15 minutes to cool.

With a spoon, dig out ⅔ of the insides of each sweet potato half to create a basket. Be careful not to break the skin.

Place the sweet potato flesh in a bowl, add onion powder and mash with a potato masher or fork.

Put the baskets back on the tray, cut side up, and press them down gently so that the bases flatten out and the baskets can stand up without wobbling.

Heat oil in a frypan over medium-low heat. Add black cumin, broccoli and carrots, and cook, stirring, for 2 minutes or until broccoli is tender but still green and crisp.

Add vegetables to the mash. Stir in cream and half the HIT-friendly Parmesan. Season with salt and pepper.

Scoop the mixture into the baskets, dividing it evenly among them. Top with the remaining HIT-friendly Parmesan.

Bake for 15-20 minutes or until they turn golden brown.

Serves 4

ZUCCHINI (COURGETTE) SLICE

> 380g (13 ounces) zucchini (courgette), grated
> 1 carrot, grated
> ¼ cup finely chopped onion
> 1/ cup olive oil
> 1 cup self-raising flour with permitted ingredients[1]
> 5 free-range egg yolks, beaten
> optional—½ cup HIT-friendly Parmesan
>   [page 110]
> salt and black pepper, according to your taste
>
> ─────────
> 1   To make self-raising flour, add 2 teaspoons of baking
> powder and ½ teaspoon salt to a cup of all-purpose flour.

Combine all ingredients and mix together well.

Pour into a greased quiche dish and bake in a moderate oven (180°C or 350 °F) until set.

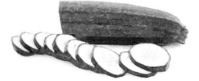

[GF] CREAMY ASPARAGUS FRITTATA

> **12 egg yolks, lightly whisked**
> **125ml (½ cup) thin cream of your choice [page 106]**
> **2 tablespoons finely chopped dill**
> **1 tablespoon rice bran oil**
> **7 tablespoons HIT-friendly butter, refrigerated, crushed to crumbs**
> **1 leek, white part only, thinly sliced**
> **2 bunches asparagus, trimmed, diagonally cut into 3cm (1 ½ inch) pieces**
> **½ teaspoon salt**
> **½ teaspoon amchoor or sumac**
> **toast and mixed salad leaves, to serve**

Preheat grill on high. Beat the egg yolks, cream and dill together in a medium bowl. Season well with salt and pepper.

Heat the rice bran oil in a large (20cm base measurement) frypan over medium heat. Add the leek and cook, stirring, for 5 minutes or until leek softens. Add the asparagus and cook, stirring, for 2 minutes or until bright green and tender but still crisp.

Pour egg mixture over the leek mixture in frypan. Gently stir to combine. Reduce heat to low and cook for 4-5 minutes or until frittata is almost set but the top is still runny. Remove from heat. Sprinkle the butter crumbs evenly over the top.

Place the frying pan under preheated grill for 2 minutes or until frittata is set and top is lightly browned.

Use a spatula to loosen the frittata and slide onto a clean work surface. Cut into wedges and place on serving plates. Serve immediately with toast and mixed salad leaves, if desired.

Serves 4

CAULIFLOWER AND BROCCOLI BAKE

> **1kg (2.2 pounds) cauliflower, cut into florets**
> **850g (3 ounces) broccoli, cut into florets**
> **3 ½ tablespoons HIT-friendly butter**
> **2 tablespoons plain (all purpose) flour with**
> **   permitted ingredients**
> **500ml (2 cups) milk of your choice [page 94]**
> **70g (1 cup) HIT-friendly Parmesan.**
> **salt and freshly ground pepper**
> **parsley to garnish**

Heat the butter in a small saucepan over medium heat until foaming but not scorching. Add the flour and cook on a low heat, stirring, for 2 minutes or until the mixture begins to bubble.

Remove from heat and slowly add milk, stirring continuously, until smooth.

Return to medium-high heat and cook, stirring, for 5 minutes or until white sauce bubbles and thickens.

Remove from heat. Stir in one-third of the HIT-friendly Parmesan. Season with salt and pepper. Cover the surface of the white sauce with non-stick baking paper (parchment paper) to prevent a skin forming, and set aside.

Steam the cauliflower and broccoli over a saucepan of boiling water for 7 minutes or until tender. Pour into a colander and allow any excess water to drain away.

Place steamed vegetable in a large, shallow, ovenproof dish.

Preheat grill to 'high'. Pour white sauce over vegetables and sprinkle with remaining HIT-friendly Parmesan.

Toast under the grill for 5 minutes or until the top is crispy, golden-brown. Serve piping hot, garnished with a few sprigs of parsley.

Serves 8

14. Salads

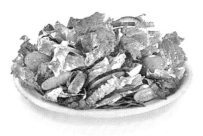

[GF] GARDEN SALAD

> 3 raw baby beetroots, juiced in a blender
> 1 cup diced, lightly steamed or blanched zucchini
>   (courgette)
> 2 cups lettuce, shredded
> 1 cucumber, thinly sliced or diced
> ½ cup roquette (aragula) leaves, shredded
> ½ cup mustard greens, chopped
> 1 mango, diced
> ½ cup ground hempseeds, for extra texture

Soak the zucchini cubes in the beetroot juice for 4 hours or overnight (refrigerated), or until they absorb the bright red color. Remove from beetroot juice and drain on paper towel. Drink or discard the beetroot juice.

Place the lettuce, mustard greens and roquette in a large serving bowl. In another bowl, mix together the mango and cucumber pieces. Spread them over the top of the shredded leaves.

Sprinkle the red-dyed zucchini on top of the salad, then sprinkle with hempseeds.

Dress with a herb oil of your choice ["Hard-Leafed Herb Oils" on page 117] and ["Soft-Leafed Herb Oils" on page 119]. Blend HIT-friendly cream with the herb oil for a creamy dressing.

You can add chopped boiled egg to this salad as a variation.

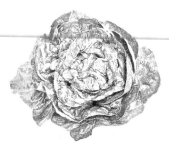

[GF] ASPARAGUS, PEA AND ROQUETTE SALAD

2 bunches asparagus, woody ends trimmed off
230g (1 ½ cups) frozen baby peas
30ml (⅛ cup) amchoor or ascorbic acid powder
3 teaspoons lemon infused oil [page 117 and
    page 119]
1 teaspoon HIT-friendly Dijon mustard ["[GF]
    HIT-friendly Dijon Mustard" on page 121]
½ teaspoon raw sugar
150g young roquette leaves

Cut the asparagus spears in half diagonally. In a steamer or microwave, steam the asparagus and peas until tender, but still green and crisp. Rinse under cold running water and allow to drain in a colander.

Beat together the lemon infused oil, HIT-friendly Dijon mustard and sugar in a small jug. Season with salt and pepper.

Place the asparagus, peas and roquette in a large serving bowl. Drizzle over the dressing and toss until well combined.

Serve straight away to preserve freshness.

Serves 6

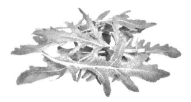

[GF] APPLESLAW

¼ (about 380g or 13 ounces) white cabbage, hard
    core removed, very thinly shredded
4 (about 500g or 18 ounces) red apples, cored,
    coarsely grated
½ small red onion, halved
finely chopped celery
½ teaspoon celery salt
1 teaspoon sumac or amchoor
1 tablespoon ascorbic acid powder
125ml (¼ cup) mascarpone
1 tablespoon ricotta
salt and freshly ground black pepper

Mix cabbage, apple, onion, celery salt, sumac and ascorbic acid powder in a bowl.

Whisk the creams or cheeses in a small bowl.

Add the creams to the cabbage mixture, and gently toss until well combined.

Taste-test, and season with salt and pepper. if required.

Pour into a serving bowl and serve immediately. Serves 6

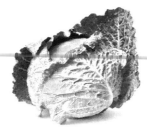

[GF] BEETROOT SALAD WITH SOFT-BOILED EGG

> **4 free-range eggs, soft-boiled and peeled**
> **½ cup HIT-friendly mayonnaise [page 122]**
> **2 teaspoons HIT-friendly Dijon mustard**
>   **[page 121]**
> **leaves from oakleaf lettuce or young cos lettuce,**
>   **roughly torn into pieces**
> **4 freshly steamed baby beetroots, cut into 2cm**
>   **(1 inch) cubes**
> **2 tablespoons chopped chives**
> **freshly ground black pepper**
> **crusty bread, to serve [page 193]**

Place the HIT-friendly mayonnaise and HIT-friendly Dijon mustard in a bowl, then add ⅓ cup (80ml or 3 fluid ounces) of boiling water. Whisk the dressing, adding a little more water if needed.

Divide the lettuce evenly between 4 serving bowls and sprinkle with the cooked beetroot.

Carefully cut in half the soft-boiled eggs, discard the white part and position the yolks on top of the beetroot. Drizzle with the dressing, season with freshly ground black pepper and garnish with chopped chives. Serve salad with crusty bread. Serves 4

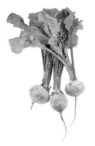

ROASTED SWEET POTATO AND BROWN RICE SALAD

750g (26 ounces) sweet potato, peeled and sliced
    into 2cm (1 inch) pieces
rice bran oil spray
1 teaspoon ground coriander (cilantro) seeds
450g (19 ounces) cooked brown rice
250g (9 ounces) broccoli, cut into small florets
½ cup parsley leaves, roughly chopped
1 red onion, thinly sliced and lightly fried
3 tablespoons pearl barley, cooked and lightly
    toasted
80ml (⅓ cup) fresh apple juice
a pinch of sumac, amchoor or ascorbic acid powder
3 teaspoons honey
½ cup shredded baby rocket leaves
50g (3 tablespoons) refrigerated HIT-friendly but-
    ter, crumbled
½ teaspoon salt

Preheat oven to 200°C. Line a baking tray with non-stick baking paper (parchment paper). Place sweet potato in a large bowl. Spray with oil. Sprinkle with coriander and toss to mix. Sprinkle with salt. Place in a single layer on tray and spray with oil. Roast for 20-25 minutes or until tender.

Place the cooked rice in a bowl and fluff it up with a fork. Allow it to cool for at least 5 minutes.

Lightly steam broccoli in a steamer or microwave, for 2-3 minutes or until just tender. Rinse under cold running water and drain. Add sweet potato, broccoli, parsley, onion and barley to rice. Whisk apple juice, sumac or ascorbic acid powder and honey in a jug until combined. Pour over rice mixture, add rocket and crumbled butter and toss to combine. Season with extra salt according to your taste.

Serves 4

[GF] CRISPY RICE NOODLE SALAD

> 4 cups shredded young wombok (Chinese cabbage)
> 4 spring onions (green onions), thinly sliced
> 1 medium carrot, peeled and grated
> 100g snow peas, thinly sliced
> ¼ cup fresh, chopped coriander leaves
> ¼ cup olive oil
> 1 tablespoon green mango juice or 1 teaspoon amchoor
> 1 tablespoon brown sugar
> 100g crunchy noodles [page 274]

Place wombok, onion, carrot, snow peas and coriander in a large bowl.

Beat oil, green mango juice and sugar together in another bowl. Pour this over cabbage mixture.

Season with salt and pepper. Toss to mix thoroughly.

Sprinkle with noodles and serve.

Serves 6

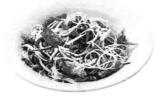

15. Side Dishes

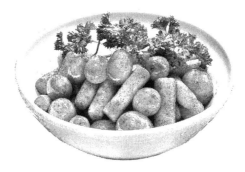

[GF] GOLDEN RICE

> **1 ½ cups water**
> **1 cup HIT-friendly milk**
> **1 ¼ cups jasmine rice or white long-grain rice**
> **1 teaspoon ground turmeric or saffron strands**

Place water and milk in a saucepan over a medium-high heat and bring to the boil. Add the rice, and the turmeric or saffron. Stir well, bring the liquid back to the boil, then turn down the heat to medium and stir again.

Cover the saucepan with a lid and simmer for 20 minutes. Remove rice from heat and allow to rest, covered, for 5 minutes. Drain through a sieve and fluff with a fork.

Serves 4

[GF] HERBED WILD RICE

> **500g (18 ounces) long-grain white rice and wild**
> **rice blend**
> **2 tablespoons fresh roughly chopped flat-leaf**
> **parsley leaves**
> **2 tablespoons fresh roughly chopped coriander**
> **(cilantro) leaves**
> **2 tablespoons fresh, chopped chives**

Cook the rice in a large saucepan of boiling, salted water following the packet instructions. Remove from the heat, drain well, then cover and keep warm until ready to serve.

Immediately before serving, pour rice into a large bowl and add the chopped fresh herbs. Toss gently to mix, and serve.

Serves 10

[GF] CARAMELIZED BROCCOLI

> **3-4 tablespoons water**
> **¼ teaspoon salt**
> **⅛ teaspoon pepper**
> **3 garlic cloves, thinly sliced (optional)**
> **3 tablespoons rice bran oil**
> **2 tablespoons green (unripe) mango juice**
> **560 g (1 ¼ lbs) broccoli, stems peeled and sliced,**
> **heads separated into small florets.**

In a large, deep frypan, heat 2 tablespoons rice bran oil on medium high, then add the broccoli stems in an even layer. Leave undisturbed for about two minutes so that they can lightly brown.

Add the florets, toss to mix and leave undisturbed for another two minutes, until the florets just start to turn brown. Toss again, cover and continue to cook over moderate heat until richly browned; about 4 minutes.

Add 3 tablespoons water, cover with a lid and cook until the broccoli is just tender and the water has evaporated; about 7 minutes. If necessary, add the spare tablespoon of water.

Pour in the last tablespoon of oil(and the garlic if you are using it) and cook, uncovered for a few more minutes until the garlic is golden brown.

Sprinkle with salt and pepper, add a dash of green mango juice and serve.

[GF] VEGETABLE CLOUDS—WHITE, ORANGE AND GREEN

White Clouds:
450g (1 pound) chopped raw cauliflower
100g chopped raw parsnip (optional)
¼ cup butter, milk, or cream of your choice
**   [page 94]**
salt and pepper
½ - 1 teaspoon garlic powder (optional)

Steam or microwave the cauliflower florets and chopped stem pieces (and parsnip if you are using it) until vegetables are tender. Test by piercing with a fork.

In a bowl or food processor, combine the remaining ingredients with the cooked vegetables. Whizz with the processor or a hand-held stick blender, until the mixture forms a smooth purée.

For orange clouds, incorporate 1 cup cooked carrot.

For green clouds, incorporate ½ cup cooked broccoli.

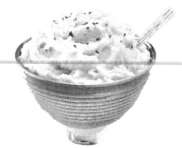

[GF] PAN-FRIED RED CABBAGE AND APPLES

> **1 Granny Smith apple, thinly sliced.**
> **1 tablespoon HIT-friendly butter**
> **1 tablespoon rice bran oil**
> **½ small red cabbage, finely shredded**
> **¼ cup apple juice**
> **½ teaspoon black cumin seeds (optional)**

On a low heat so as not to scorch the butter, melt butter and oil in a large non-stick frypan. Add the apple slices and cook, frequently flipping them over, for 3 to 4 minutes or until pale gold in color. Transfer to a plate.

Add cabbage, juice and black cumin seeds to frypan and stir to blend. Cook, while gently tossing the pan, for 3 minutes or until cabbage is barely wilted. Stir the apples through the cabbage mixture. Season with salt and pepper and serve.

Serves 4

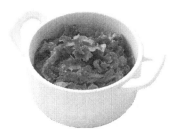

[GF] MAPLE SPICE CANDIED SWEET POTATOES

> **100g (2 pounds) sweet potatoes, preferably with colored flesh**
> **¼ cup HIT-friendly butter**
> **¼ cup maple syrup**
> **⅓ cup packed brown sugar**
> **¼ teaspoon ground cardamom or allspice**

In a large saucepan, cover sweet potatoes with water and bring to a boil.

Lower heat and simmer for 25 minutes, until sweet potatoes are tender.

Remove from saucepan and allow to cool. When cooled, peel and cut into wedges.

Place in 2 liter (2 quart) baking dish.

In small saucepan combine remaining ingredients, cook and stir until mixture boils.

Pour sugar and spice mixture over sweet potatoes.

Bake at 180°C (350°F) for 40 minutes.

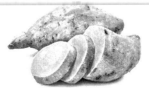

16. Breads

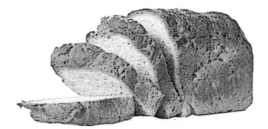

WHEAT-FREE FLOUR BLENDS FOR BAKING

Wheat-free, gluten-free flour blends are widely available in stores. If you prefer to make your own, here are two basic blends you can keep on hand for baking. Store in an airtight container in a cool, dark place and make small batches at a time, so that it will be used while still fresh.

[GF] SIMPLE GLUTEN-FREE FLOUR BLEND

1 cup oat flour or brown rice flour
1 cup cornstarch
½ cup millet flour
1 teaspoon guar gum

Combine all ingredients.
This blend is useful for baking breads, muffins, cookies, cakes and cupcakes.

[GF] RICH GLUTEN-FREE FLOUR BLEND

1 cup oat flour or brown rice flour
1 cup cornstarch
½ cup millet flour
½ cup cornmeal
¼ cup water-chestnut flour
1.5 teaspoons guar gum OR 1.5 teaspoons chia seeds, (later to be whisked with 3 teaspoons boiling water).

Combine all ingredients (except chia seeds if you are using them, which must be kept separate).
This is a slightly richer blend, useful for baking everything.

BAKING HINTS

Hint #1: You can add ¼ cup hempseed meal to your flour blend for added fiber.

Hint #2: If you find your baked products are too crumbly, increase guar gum by a small amount, e.g. by ⅛ – ¼ teaspoon at a time.

Hint #3: As a replacement for guar gum in recipes, you can use chia seeds. Substitute the same quantity of chia seeds, whisked briskly with twice as much boiling water to form a slurry. Then add it to your other ingredients.

Hint #4: Eggs are useful for thickening and binding in baking, but you may wish to replace them.
One egg = 1 tablespoon finely ground chia seeds whipped with ¼ cup water. The chia seeds form a gel and bind with the other ingredients.

Hint #5: Other egg replacements include applesauce, or puréed summer squash (yellow patty-pan squash), or zucchini (courgette).
These substitutes will bind ingredients together, as egg does. They are low in fat and will also contribute some flavor, so choose your egg replacer according to how you want the recipe to turn out. 1 egg = ¼ cup purée.

Hint #6: The best milks for baking are those which contain some fat. For example, rice milk is useful for cooking, but used in baking it makes products that are rather dry, instead of rich and satisfying. Oat milk is good for baking.

Hint #7: To make self-raising flour, add 2 teaspoons of baking powder and ½ teaspoon salt to a cup of all-purpose flour.

ABOUT SODA BREAD

Soda bread (Irish: arán sóide, Scots: fardel) is a quickly-made bread traditional to many cuisines; most famously, Irish and Scots.

It gets its English name from the fact that it's made using sodium bicarbonate (otherwise known as baking soda) as a leavening agent, instead of yeast.

'The ingredients of traditional soda bread are flour, bread soda, salt, and buttermilk. The buttermilk in the dough contains lactic acid, which reacts with the baking soda to form tiny bubbles of carbon dioxide.' [217]

[GF] SIMPLE SODA BREAD

> **500g (17.5 ounces) plain all-purpose gluten free flour with permitted ingredients [page 194], plus a little extra for sprinkling**
> **1 teaspoon bicarb soda (baking soda)**
> **½ teaspoon salt**
> **310ml (10 fluid ounces) buttermilk [page 99]**
> **rice bran oil spray**

Preheat oven to 200° C (400° F). Grease a baking tray with rice bran oil spray.

Sift flour, bicarb soda and salt into a mixing bowl. Make a hollow in the middle of the dry ingredients and pour in the buttermilk. With a wooden spoon, gently stir the ingredients until they are well mixed and form a soft dough.

Wet your hands with cold water to stop the dough from sticking to them. Scrape the dough together with your fingers, then tip it out onto a clean surface such as a large wooden chopping board, sprinkled lightly with flour. Lightly knead it until it is smooth and shape it into a sphere.

Put dough on baking tray and flatten it a little to form a round, domed loaf about 19 cm (7.5 inches) in diameter.

Take a sharp knife and cut a deep cross in the top, slicing half-way down into the dough. Sprinkle extra flour over the top.

Place tray in preheated oven and bake for about 30 minutes or until the loaf has risen well, the top is brown and the bread sounds hollow when you tap it. If it seems undercooked, give it another 3–5 minutes in the oven and then test again.

When baked, remove loaf from oven and place on a wire rack. Allow it to cool thoroughly before cutting slices.

Serve as an accompaniment to soups and stews.

Use bread on the day it is baked. Soda bread is delicious when fresh, but becomes stale quite rapidly. If this happens, simply toast it. It is best stored sliced, in the freezer.

Serves: 8

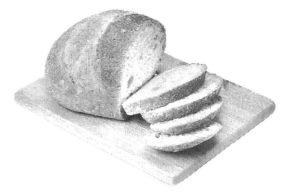

RICH SODA BREAD

4 cups plain flour with permitted ingredients
4 tablespoons white sugar
1 teaspoon baking soda
1 tablespoon baking powder
½ teaspoon salt
½ cup HIT-friendly butter, softened
1 cup buttermilk [page 99]
1 free-range egg
3 tablespoons HIT-friendly butter, melted
¼ cup extra buttermilk

Preheat oven to 180° C (350 ° F). Lightly grease a large baking tray with rice bran oil spray.

In a large bowl, mix together flour, sugar, baking soda, baking powder, salt and butter. After they are well blended, stir in 1 cup of buttermilk and the egg.

Mix to form a dough. Turn dough out onto a lightly floured surface and knead lightly. Form dough into a round loaf and place on greased baking tray.

In a small bowl, combine melted butter with extra buttermilk. Dip in a pastry brush and brush the top of the loaf with this mixture so that it will turn golden-brown when baked. Use a sharp knife to cut a deep cross into the top of the loaf.

Bake loaf in preheated oven for 45 to 50 minutes, or until the loaf sounds hollow when tapped with your fingers. You may continue to brush the loaf with the butter mixture while it bakes.

Remove from oven and allow to cool on a wire rack. Soda bread is best eaten on the day of baking. To store, cut into slices and freeze in freezer bags. Warm or toast the slices when you need to use them. Serves: 20

[GF] MESOPOTAMIAN HEMP BREAD

Since this bread contains no yeast, nuts or wheat, HIT sufferers can enjoy it freely.

---

1 ⅓ cups hempseed meal
⅔ cup water-chestnut flour
3 teaspoons baking powder
½ teaspoon salt (or to taste)
1 ½ tablespoons olive oil
4 free-range egg yolks
rice bran oil spray
rock salt or salt flakes for topping (optional)
water (approx. 2 tablespoons)

Preheat oven to 180° C (350° F). Grease a bread loaf tin with oil spray, line it with baking paper (parchment paper) and grease the baking paper.

In a bowl, thoroughly mix together the dry ingredients. In a separate bowl, lightly whisk the egg yolks. Pour yolks into dry ingredients.

Add water gradually, mixing well, until the batter reaches your desired texture. Use the least amount of water possible. If the batter is too wet, the loaf will not cook all the way through.

Paint the top of the loaf with water and sprinkle with coarse salt if desired. Place loaf tin in the oven and bake for approximately 20 – 25 minutes or until golden brown on top. Test whether it is cooked inside by inserting a metal skewer or butter knife into the middle of the loaf. If it comes out clean, the bread is ready.

Take it out of the oven and allow it to rest for 5 -10 minutes before turning it out of the tin onto a wire rack.

Serve warm, straight out of the oven or cold for sandwiches.

For variations, try adding a tablespoon of finely chopped sage or rosemary, or a teaspoon of chopped oregano and some pepper, or chopped spring onions (green onions) or broccoli.

For sweet bread add cardamom, honey and chopped, dried mango.

[GF] STONE AGE BREAD #1

Deliciously yeast-free, nut-free, dairy-free and wheat-free.

> 2 cups water-chestnut flour
> 2 tablespoons arrowroot
> ¼ cup hempseed meal
> ¼ teaspoon salt
> ½ teaspoon baking soda
> 5 free-range egg yolks
> 1 tablespoon HIT-friendly oil
> 1 tablespoon honey
> 1 tablespoon green (unripe) mango juice [page
>   116] or ½ tablespoon amchoor [page 114]
> rice bran oil spray

Preheat oven to 180° C (350°F). Grease a 20 x 9cm (7.5 x 3.5 inch) loaf tin with rice bran oil spray, line it with baking paper (parchment paper) and oil the baking paper.

Place water-chestnut flour, arrowroot, hempseed meal, salt and baking soda in a food processor. Using short bursts of power, 'pulse' them until they are mixed.

Add egg yolks, oil, honey and green mango juice or amchoor, and again 'pulse' to blend.

Pour the batter into the greased loaf tin, place it in the oven and bake for 30 minutes until cooked through. Remove from oven and allow to cool for 5 - 10 minutes.

Turn out loaf onto a wire rack, cool and serve.

[GF] STONE AGE BREAD #2

> **4 to 5 free-range egg yolks**
> **⅔ cup hempseed meal**
> **1⅓ cup water-chestnut flour**
> **1½ - 2 teaspoons baking powder**
> **½ teaspoon salt, or more, to taste**
> **2 tablespoon olive oil**
> **rice bran oil spray**

Preheat oven to 180° C (350°F). Grease a loaf tin with rice bran oil spray, line it with baking paper (parchment paper) and oil the baking paper.

Place egg yolks into a large bowl, lightly beat them and then add dry ingredients. Mix thoroughly.

Pour batter into greased loaf tin. It is a thick batter, so use a spoon to spread it evenly in the tin and smooth out the surface.

Bake for 20 – 25 minutes, until lightly-browned on top. Test whether it is cooked inside by inserting a metal skewer or butter knife into the middle of the loaf. If it comes out clean, the bread is ready.

Remove from oven and allow to cool for 5 - 10 minutes.

Turn out loaf onto a wire rack, cool and serve warm or cold. Store any leftover bread in refrigerator to keep it fresh, or freeze in slices for later use.

[GF] HIT-FRIENDLY SANDWICH BREAD

¾ cup tapioca flour, sifted
¼ cup hempseed meal
2 tablespoons arrowroot
½ teaspoons baking soda
1 teaspoons baking powder
¾ teaspoon salt
1 teaspoon onion powder
⅛ cup black cumin seeds (plus 1 tablespoon)
7 free-range egg yolks, beaten
½ cup melted HIT-friendly butter
2 tablespoons HIT-friendly sour cream or plain
    cream

Preheat oven to 160° C (325°F). Grease a loaf tin with rice bran oil spray, line it with baking paper (parchment paper) and oil the baking paper.

In a bowl, mix together the arrowroot, baking soda, baking powder, salt, onion powder and ⅛ cup black cumin seeds.

In another bowl, beat together the egg yolks and sour cream or other HIT-friendly cream.

Pour the egg mixture into the bowl of dry ingredients and stir well. Then add the melted butter and mix until thoroughly combined.

Pour batter into loaf tin, sprinkle with the extra black cumin seeds and place tin in preheated oven.

Bake 40-50 minutes. Test whether it is cooked inside by inserting a metal skewer or butter knife into the middle of the loaf. If it comes out clean, the bread is ready.

Remove from oven and allow to cool for 5 - 10 minutes. Turn out loaf onto a wire rack, cool and serve warm or cold.

Store any leftover bread in refrigerator to keep it fresh, or freeze in slices for later use.

FIVE FLOURS BREAD

A versatile bread recipe suitable for making moist, tender and cushiony dinner rolls, pizza crust or sandwich bread.

Contains no yeast, eggs or wheat.

2 tablespoons ground hemp meal
6 tablespoons boiling water
⅓ cup millet flour, sifted
¼ cup brown rice flour, sifted
¼ cup cornstarch, sifted
½ cup arrowroot flour, sifted
2 teaspoon baking powder
1 teaspoon baking soda
¾ teaspoon salt
1 teaspoon guar gum
1 tablespoon honey
2 tablespoons olive oil
½ cup HIT-friendly cream
2 tablespoons cold water
1 tablespoon green mango juice or ½ tablespoon
    amchoor
rice bran oil spray

Preheat oven to 190° C (375°F). Grease a baking tray with rice bran oil spray, line it with baking paper (parchment paper) and oil the baking paper.

In a small mixing bowl, stir together the hempseed meal and boiling water. Set aside and allow to stand for 10 minutes.

In another bowl, mix together the flours, baking powder, soda, salt, and guar gum.

Using a third bowl, thoroughly combine the honey, oil, HIT-friendly cream, water, and green mango juice (or amchoor). Pour in the hemp mixture and stir well.

Now gradually pour the bowl of wet ingredients into the bowl of dry ingredients, stirring until barely blended.

Divide the dough into two equal portions, scoop each portion out of the bowl, shape them into rounds about 15cm (6 inches) in diameter and place them on opposite sides of the baking tray.

Place in preheated oven and bake for 20 – 25 minutes.

Test whether loaves are cooked inside by inserting a metal skewer or butter knife into the middle. If it comes out clean, the bread is ready.

Remove from oven and allow to cool for 5 - 10 minutes.

Turn out loaves onto a wire rack and allow to cool further before slicing.

Store any leftover bread in refrigerator to keep it fresh, or freeze in slices for later use.

For sandwiches, slice loaves horizontally to get a large surface area.

For pizza crust, add 1 to 2 teaspoons of Italian seasoning ["Home Made Italian Seasoning" on page 118] and 1 clove of crushed garlic to the dough. Using a wet spatula, spread out the dough on a baking tray, as evenly as possible. Bake for about 10 minutes, or more if needed. Remove from oven and cover with HIT-friendly pizza toppings such as herbs, egg, roasted vegetables and seasonings. Bake for another 10 to 20 minutes.

For dinner rolls, add a teaspoon of chopped chives or rosemary to the dough, then separate into 6 to 8 rounds. Top with black cumin seeds and bake for 10 – 15 minutes.

[GF] SOFT AND SPRINGY CORNBREAD

2 cups cornmeal
2 teaspoons baking powder
¼ teaspoon bicarbonate of soda
2 cups buttermilk ["About Buttermilk" on page 97]
1 large free-range egg, beaten
1 tablespoon sugar
½ teaspoon salt
⅓ cup rice bran oil
rice bran oil spray

Preheat oven to 220°C (425°F). Using the ⅓ cup oil, grease the base and inner sides of a 25cm (10 inch) diameter round metal baking tin or cast-iron ovenproof frypan.

In a large bowl, sift together the cornmeal, baking powder and bicarbonate of soda and combine well.

Stir in the buttermilk, egg, salt and sugar.

Pour cornbread batter into the oiled ovenproof dish and set the dish in the oven.

Bake for 25 minutes or until golden-brown on top. When cornbread is ready, turn it out of the baking tin straight away and allow it to cool on a wire rack. Serve as a side dish or a snack.

Serves 6 to 8.

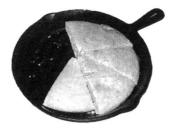

[GF] CORNBREAD WITH SOUR CREAM

425g (15 ounces) fresh or frozen sweetcorn
    kernels
1 cup sour cream ["[GF] Hit-Friendly Sour
    Cream" on page 105]
2 free-range egg yolks, beaten
¼ cup HIT-friendly butter, melted
1 cup cornmeal
1 teaspoons baking powder
⅛ teaspoon bicarbonate of soda
1 tablespoon sugar or sweetener of your choice
    [page 86]
2 tablespoons unsweetened applesauce or
    apple purée
rice bran oil spray

Preheat oven to 190° C (375° F). Oil a 22 x 12 cm (9 x 5 inches) loaf tin with rice bran oil spray, line it with baking paper (parchment paper) and oil the baking paper.

In a large bowl, combine sweetcorn kernels, sour cream, egg yolks and melted butter. Slowly mix in the cornmeal, baking powder, bicarbonate of soda, sugar and applesauce.

When all is thoroughly combined, pour the batter into the prepared tin and place in the oven.

Bake for 25 minutes. Test whether loaf is cooked through by inserting a metal skewer or butter knife into the center. If it comes out clean, the bread is ready.

For a variation, you could add onion powder or finely chopped onions to the mixture.

[GF] TASTY CORNBREAD WITH BROCCOLI

2 free-range egg yolks
1 cup (8 ounces) whipped cream of your choice
3 cups frozen chopped broccoli, thawed
¾ cup finely chopped onion
6 tablespoons HIT-friendly butter, melted
510g (18 ounces) cornmeal
2 teaspoons baking powder
1 teaspoon baking soda
rice bran oil spray

Preheat oven to 180° C (350° F). Grease the base and inner sides of a 25cm (10 inch) diameter round metal baking tin or cast-iron ovenproof frypan with rice bran oil spray, line it with baking paper (parchment paper) and oil the baking paper.

In a mixing bowl, lightly beat egg yolks. Add whipped cream, broccoli, onion, melted butter, cornmeal, baking soda and baking powder. Beat well until thoroughly combined.

Pour batter into ovenproof container. Bake for 40-45 minutes or until golden-brown. When cornbread is ready, turn it out of the baking tin straight away and allow it to cool a little on a wire rack.

Cut into wedges and serve warm.

Serves 12-16.

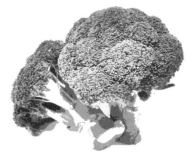

YEAST-FREE CIABATTA

'Ciabatta (literally 'slipper bread') is an Italian white bread made from wheat flour and yeast, created in 1982 by a baker in Italy, in response to the popularity of French baguettes. Ciabatta is somewhat elongated, broad and flat and is baked in many variations.' [218]

> 3 cups plain (all-purpose) flour with permitted ingredients
> 5 teaspoons baking powder
> 1/2 teaspoon salt
> 1 1/2 tablespoons olive oil
> water
> toasted rolled oats for scattering over the top of the loaf
> rice bran oil spray

Preheat oven to 200°C (400°F). Grease a baking tray with rice bran oil spray.

Mix together the flour, baking powder and salt. Stir in the oil and enough water to make a firm, smooth dough that is not over-sticky.

Pat the dough into a long, low, rectangular shape and put it on the baking tray.

Wet your fingers, paint the water over the top of the loaf and sprinkle with toasted rolled oats. Gently press in the oats, then lightly powder the loaf with white flour.

Place in the oven and bake for about 20 minutes or until golden-brown.

[GF] YEAST-FREE, WHEAT-FREE CRUSTY BREAD

This bread is suitable for making Italian ciabatta, French baguettes and breadsticks. You can make it in a specially-shaped French bread pan or in a loaf tin.

> 1 3/4 cups (185 grams or 6.5 ounces) water-chestnut flour
> 5 teaspoons hempseed meal
> 3 teaspoons baking powder
> 1 teaspoon salt
> 1 tablespoon sugar or honey
> 2 tablespoons green mango juice (or unripe apple juice, preferably with a pinch of amchoor, page 114)
> 2 medium free-range egg yolks, beaten
> 1/2 cup boiling water
> rice bran oil spray

Preheat oven to 180° C (350° F). Grease a bread loaf tin or French bread pan with rice bran oil spray, line it with baking paper (parchment paper) and grease the baking paper.

In a medium bowl, beat the water-chestnut flour, hempseed meal, baking powder, and salt.

Beat the sugar, green mango juice or unripe apple juice and egg yolks in a small bowl. Add the sugar mixture to the large bowl and stir, using a large spoon.

Pour in the boiling water and mix well until the dough comes together. It will still be rather sticky -that's normal.

Scoop the dough out of the bowl and into the loaf pan. Pour a little rice bran oil into your hand and stroke it over the top of the dough, shaping it into a loaf.

Bake for one hour or until the internal temperature is 88 - 94°C (190-200°F). Do not overcook. If you have a cooking thermometer, insert it into the loaf when you think it is done, to check.

When the bread is ready remove it from the oven and turn it out onto a wire rack to cool.

Makes one loaf.

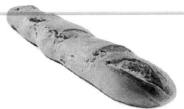

17. Cakes, Muffins & Cookies

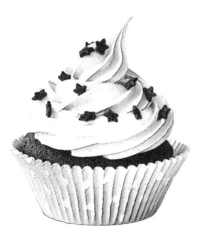

HELPFUL BAKING HINTS

For basic make-your-own flour mixes see ["Wheat-Free Flour Blends For Baking" on page 194], and for handy tips, see ["Baking Hints" on page 195.]

APPLE CAKE

> **125g HIT-friendly butter, chilled and chopped**
> **½ cup firmly packed brown sugar**
> **1 teaspoon natural, oil-based vanilla essence**
> **2 free-range egg yolks**
> **1 cup self-raising flour with permitted ingredients[1]**
> **½ cup plain (all-purpose) flour with permitted ingredients**
> **¾ cup oat milk [page 94]**
> **2 small cooking apples**
> **¼ cup fig jam or other HIT-friendly jam of your choice ["Jams, Jellies & Preserves" on page 229]**
> **rice bran oil spray**
> **sweetened, whipped HIT-friendly cream, to serve**
>
> ---
> 1   To make self-raising flour, sift 2 teaspoons of baking powder and ¼ teaspoon bicarbonate of soda (baking soda)into 1 cup all-purpose flour and mix well.

Preheat oven to 180°C (350° F). For fan-forced ovens, as a general rule, the oven temperature should be set 20°C (68°F) lower.

Spray oil around the inside of a 6cm (2.5 inches)-deep, 20cm (8 inch) diameter circular spring-form baking tin. Line base with baking paper (parchment paper) and spray paper with more oil.

Put butter, sugar and vanilla in the bowl of an electric mixer. Beat for 5 to 6 minutes or until light and creamy.

Add egg yolks, one at a time, beating after each addition.

Sift flours over butter mixture. Add milk and fold it through until all ingredients are just barely combined. Scoop cake mixture into prepared baking tin.

Remove cores from apples and cut them into quarters. Thinly slice them and arrange the slices in two circles on top of the cake mixture, gently pressing them into place.

Bake for 35 to 40 minutes or until a metal skewer inserted in the middle comes out clean.

Remove from oven and allow cake to rest in the tin for 10 minutes. Unclasp the walls of the tin and slide cake onto a wire rack to cool.

Spoon the jam into a microwave-safe bowl. Microwave on high (100%) for 30 seconds to 1 minute or until runny. Brush cake top with jam. Serve with whipped HIT-friendly cream.

Serves 8

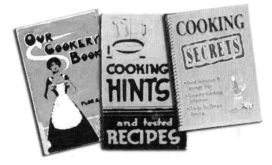

APPLE GALETTE

A galette is a flat, round French-style cake usually made with flaky or puff pastry.

**1 25 x 25cm (9.5 x 9.5 inches) puff pastry sheet—
    preferably wheat free[1]
2 large Granny Smith apples, peeled, thinly sliced
2 tablespoons melted HIT-friendly butter
2 tablespoons caster sugar
rice bran oil spray
honey, to serve**

---

1   Frozen, gluten free puff pastry is widely available
in stores. Check labels for permitted ingredients.

Preheat the oven to 180°C (350°F). Lightly grease a baking tray with rice bran oil.

Cut four 12cm (4.5 inches) circles from the puff pastry. Lay them on the tray.

Decoratively position the apples slices, overlapping, on top of the pastry. Brush with melted butter and sprinkle with sugar.

Bake for 20-25 minutes until the pastry is golden-brown and crispy. Serve warm, drizzled with honey.

Serves 4

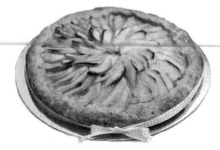

[GF] APPLE TEA CAKE

2 firm cooking-apples such as Granny Smith
2 tablespoons green mango juice or (unripe apple
**   juice with a pinch of amchoor, page 114)**
2 teaspoon ground cardamom
250g caster sugar
250g HIT-friendly butter, unsalted
1 ⅔ cup (250g) gluten free self-raising flour with
**   permitted ingredients[1] [page 194]**
4 free-range egg yolks
icing sugar, to dust
rice bran oil spray

---

1   To make self-raising flour from all-purpose flour see Hint #7, page 195.

Preheat oven to 180°C (350°F). For fan-forced ovens, as a general rule, the oven temperature should be set 20°C (68°F) lower.

Use rice bran oil spray to grease a 23cm (9 inch) springform cake pan, then line the base with baking paper (parchment paper).

Peel and core the apples, cut into quarters, then cut each quarter into thin slices. Toss the apples in green mango juice and half the cardamom, then set aside.

Take 50g (1 ½ ounces) each of the sugar, butter and flour, place in a bowl with the remaining cardamom and rub together with your fingertips until the mixture resembles crumbs.

Place egg yolks and remaining sugar in an electric mixer and beat until very light and fluffy. Melt remaining butter and pour into egg mixture. Sift in remaining flour, then fold in gently until combined.

Pour into the pan, and decoratively lay the apple slices over top. Sprinkle with the crumble mixture and bake for 50 minutes or until a skewer inserted into the center comes out clean.

Allow to cool for 10 minutes before transferring to a wire rack to cool completely. Serve dusted with icing sugar.

Serves 8

[GF] CARDAMOM SHORTBREAD

rice bran oil, to grease
250g (9 ounces) HIT-friendly butter, unsalted, at
    room temperature
125g (4 ½ ounces) brown sugar
1 teaspoon natural caramel flavor ["[GF] Caramel
    Essence" on page 128]
190g (6 ½ ounces) gluten free plain flour with
    permitted ingredients [page 194]
135g (5 ounces) rice flour
1 ½ teaspoon ground cardamom or allspice
icing sugar mixture, to dust

Preheat oven to 150°C (300°F). Lightly grease two 8.5 x 25cm (3.5 x 8 inch) bar pans by brushing with rice bran oil. Line base and 2 long sides with non-stick baking paper (parchment paper), allowing sides to overhang.

Use an electric mixer to beat together the butter, sugar and caramel until well combined.

Place the gluten free plain flour, the rice flour and the spice in a bowl and stir to blend. Sift the blended flours and spice over the butter mixture. Use a wooden spoon to stir until well mixed.

Divide the dough into 2 portions. Press 1 portion into each of the prepared pans. Score the shortbread crossways, about 1cm deep, into 12 even pieces.

Place in oven and bake for 50 minutes or until lightly browned.

Remove pans from oven and allow them to cool down for 30 minutes before turning out the shortbread onto a wire rack to cool completely. Dust with icing sugar to serve.

Serves: 24

JAM SURPRISE MUFFINS

250g (9 ounces) plain flour with permitted
  ingredients
1 tablespoon baking powder
½ teaspoon bicarbonate of soda
2 tablespoons caster sugar
2 tablespoons brown sugar
60g (2 ounces) HIT-friendly butter, unsalted,
  melted and cooled
½ tablespoon mango amchoor [page 114]
250ml (8 fluid ounces) buttermilk [page 99]
1 free-range egg, lightly beaten
½ cup fig jam ["[GF] Fig Jam" on page 235]
2 fresh figs, sliced
icing sugar, to dust

Preheat the oven to 200°C (400°F). You will need a muffin tray with 12 pans. If you use a silicone muffin tray, you won't need to grease the pans. If using a metal muffin tray, line it with baking paper (parchment paper) squares or muffin cases.

If you use squares, cut pieces of baking paper each about 13cm (5 inches) square. Grease the muffin pans, and line them with the squares. Allow the paper to extend above the sides of the muffin pans to support the muffins as they rise.

Sift flour, baking powder, bicarbonate of soda, caster sugar, brown sugar and ½ teaspoon salt into a large bowl. In a separate bowl, combine the melted butter, amchoor, buttermilk and egg.

Add egg mixture to dry ingredients, then with a large spoon or spatula, fold together until barely combined.

Spoon 2 tablespoonsful of muffin batter into the base of each muffin pan. Add 2 teaspoonsful of fig jam to each, then fill with the remaining batter. Top each muffin with a slice of fig.

Bake the muffins for 18-20 minutes until light golden brown and a metal skewer inserted in the center comes out clean.

Dust with icing sugar and serve. Serves: 12

MINI FIG MUFFINS WITH CARAMEL FUDGE SAUCE

Mini Fig Muffins:
melted butter or rice bran oil, to grease
250g (9 ounces) fresh figs, finely chopped
125ml (4 fluid ounces) water
2 teaspoons finely grated fresh ginger
1 teaspoon bicarbonate of soda
300g (10.5 ounces) self-raising flour with permitted ingredients
155g (5 ounces) brown sugar
125ml (4 fluid ounces) olive oil
2 free-range egg yolks, lightly whisked

Caramel Fudge Sauce:
80g (3 ounces) HIT-friendly butter
125ml (4 fluid ounces) thick, whipped HIT-friendly cream
100g (3.5 ounces) brown sugar
1 tablespoon golden syrup

Preheat oven to 180°C (350°F). Brush twelve 40ml (2-tablespoons) capacity mini muffin pans with melted butter or rice bran oil, to grease.

Put the chopped figs and the water in a medium-sized saucepan over a medium heat and bring to the boil.

Remove from heat, then add the ginger and bicarbonate of soda and mix until blended. Allow the mixture to stand for 10 minutes to cool down.

Put the flour and sugar into a mixing bowl. With a large spoon, stir in the fig mixture, olive oil and egg until well combined.

Spoon one-quarter of the mixture evenly among the prepared mini muffin pans. Place the tray in the oven and bake for 12-15 minutes or until a metal skewer inserted into the centers of the muffins comes out clean.

Turn out the muffins onto a wire rack to cool. Repeat, in 3 more batches, with the remaining mixture, brushing the pans with rice bran oil or melted butter to grease between batches.

To make the caramel fudge sauce, combine the butter, cream, sugar and golden syrup in a medium saucepan over medium heat. Cook, stirring, for 2-3 minutes or until all ingredients have melted together to form a smooth sauce.

Pile muffins on a platter. Drizzle the sauce over them to serve.

Serves: 8

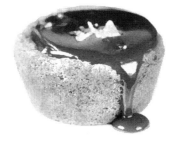

[GF] AUSTRIAN VANILLA CRESCENTS

Austrian *vanillekipferl* are festive delicacies usually eaten at Christmas time, and made with almonds or other nuts. Here is the HIT-friendly version.

Dusting and homemade vanilla sugar:
115g sugar
½ vanilla bean

Vanilla Crescents:
170g (6 ounces) plain (all-purpose) gluten free
    flour with permitted ingredients [page 194]
65g (just over 2 ounces) cornstarch
55g (just under 2 ounces) sugar
2 free-range egg yolks
125g (4 ½ ounces) HIT-friendly butter
rice bran oil spray

Preheat oven to 175°C (80°F). Spray a baking tray with rice bran oil.

Vanilla sugar:

Place the 115g sugar and the ½ vanilla bean into a food processor and process on high speed until well mixed. You now have homemade vanilla sugar.

Place into a mixing bowl the flour, cornstarch, sugar, 1 tablespoon homemade vanilla sugar, egg yolks and butter.

Mix well, then knead with your hands to form a dough. Cover the bowl of dough with plastic wrap and chill for 1 hour in the refrigerator.

Remove from refrigerator and form into small crescents weighing about 14g (½ ounce) each.

Place the crescents on the oiled tray and bake for 12 minutes. Remove from oven, allow to cool a little, then and roll them in the remaining vanilla sugar while they are still warm.

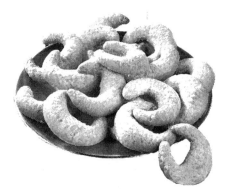

LIGHT AND MOIST LAVENDER CUPCAKES

Lavender oil has been demonstrated to inhibit histamine release. [219] Lavender is edible, but you must select culinary-quality flowers—those that have never been sprayed with pesticides. Do not eat lavender bought from a florist or nursery. Pick your own or buy from a specialized spice shop.

Note: the preparation begins the night before!

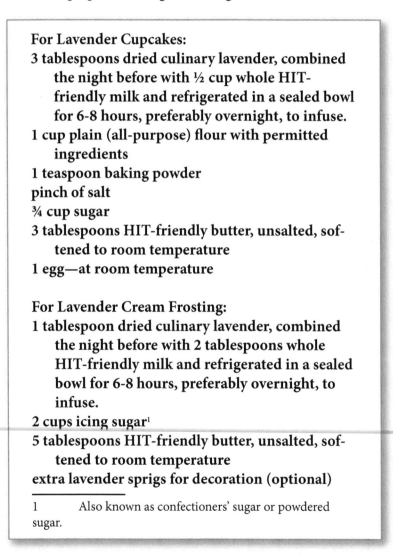

For Lavender Cupcakes:
3 tablespoons dried culinary lavender, combined the night before with ½ cup whole HIT-friendly milk and refrigerated in a sealed bowl for 6-8 hours, preferably overnight, to infuse.
1 cup plain (all-purpose) flour with permitted ingredients
1 teaspoon baking powder
pinch of salt
¾ cup sugar
3 tablespoons HIT-friendly butter, unsalted, softened to room temperature
1 egg—at room temperature

For Lavender Cream Frosting:
1 tablespoon dried culinary lavender, combined the night before with 2 tablespoons whole HIT-friendly milk and refrigerated in a sealed bowl for 6-8 hours, preferably overnight, to infuse.
2 cups icing sugar[1]
5 tablespoons HIT-friendly butter, unsalted, softened to room temperature
extra lavender sprigs for decoration (optional)

---

1   Also known as confectioners' sugar or powdered sugar.

Preheat oven to 160°C (325°F). Prepare a cupcake tray by inserting cupcake liners of your choice.

To Make Lavender Cupcakes:

Using a fine sieve, strain the infused milk into a jug, to remove the lavender flowers. Set jug aside.

Into the bowl of an electric mixer, sift together the flour, baking powder and salt.

Add the sugar and softened butter to the dry ingredients and beat at a low speed until all ingredients are combined and the texture is crumbly.

Keep the beating speed on low while you gradually pour the infused milk from the jug into the flour mixture. When the last of the milk is blended, turn off the mixer and add the egg.

Now beat for 15 seconds on medium speed, then scrape down the sides and the bottom of the bowl with a spatula, to make certain all ingredients are well-mixed. Be careful not to overmix, or you will end up with dry cupcakes.

Spoon batter into the cupcake liners until they are two thirds full. Set the cupcake tray in the oven and bake for 20-23 minutes or until an inserted metal skewer comes out clean.

Transfer cupcakes to a wire cooling rack and leave until completely cool.

To Make Lavender Cream Frosting:

Using a fine sieve, strain the infused milk into a jug, to remove the lavender flowers. Set jug aside.

Sift icing sugar into the bowl of an electric mixer and add the softened butter. Beat on low speed until combined.

Keep the beating speed on low while you gradually pour in the infused milk. When butter and sugar are well combined, increase beating speed to high for 5 minutes until frosting is light and fluffy. Optional: if you have any HIT friendly food colorings such as "[GF] Purple Or Blue Food Dyes" on page 128, you can add them at this stage.

Slather the cooled cupcakes with frosting and top with tiny sprigs of lavender flowers, to decorate. Serves: 10—12 cupcakes.

[GF] CHEWY SPICE COOKIES

2¼ cups plain (all-purpose) gluten free flour with
   permitted ingredients [page 194]
1 teaspoon baking soda
1½ teaspoons ground cardamom
1½ teaspoons ground ginger
¾ teaspoon ground allspice
¼ teaspoon ground black pepper
¼ teaspoon salt
¾ cup HIT-friendly butter, unsalted, at room
   temperature
⅓ cup sugar
⅓ cup dark brown sugar
1 free-range egg yolk
1 teaspoon natural vanilla extract
½ cup molasses
½ cup sugar (extra for rolling)

Preheat oven to 375 degrees F. Line two baking sheets with baking paper (parchment paper).

In a medium bowl, whisk together the flour, baking soda, cinnamon, ginger, cloves, allspice, pepper and salt; set aside.

Using an electric mixer, beat together the butter and both sugars on medium-high speed until light and fluffy, about 3 minutes. Reduce the speed to medium-low, add the egg yolk and vanilla extract, increase the speed to medium and beat until thoroughly combined, about 30 seconds.

Again reduce the speed to medium-low and add the molasses, beating until fully incorporated, about 30 seconds, scraping the sides of the bowl halfway through. Reduce the speed to low and gradually add the dry ingredients, mixing until just incorporated, about 30 seconds. Use a rubber spatula to give it a final few mixes to ensure no flour remains.

Place the sugar for rolling in a small bowl. Using a tablespoon or small cookie scoop, scoop the dough and roll into a smooth ball, then toss in the sugar to coat and place on the prepared baking sheet. Repeat with the remaining dough. Bake the cookies, one sheet at a time, until the cookies are browned, still puffy and the edges have begun to set but the centers are still soft, about 11 minutes. Be sure not to overbake the cookies.

Allow the cookies to cool on the baking sheet for 5 minutes, then remove to a wire rack to cool completely. The cookies can be stored in an airtight container at room temperature for up to 5 days.

These warm, chewy cookies are full of spice and the perfect accompaniment to a cup of coffee or tea.

Yield: About 24 cookies

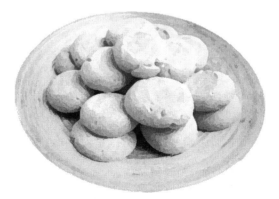

[GF] MILLET BLOSSOM COOKIES

> **125g (4 ounces) HIT-friendly butter**
> **½ cup sugar**
> **1 teaspoon vanilla extract**
> **1 free-range egg**
> **1 ¼ cups gluten free self-raising flour with permitted ingredients, sifted[1] [page 194]**
> **1 cup puffed millet**
> **1 ½ cups corn flakes, crushed**
>
> ---
>
> 1   To make self-raising flour from all-purpose flour see Hint #7, page 195.

Preheat oven to 180°C (350°F). Line a baking tray with non-stick baking paper (parchment paper).

Place butter, sugar and vanilla extract into the bowl of an electric mixer and beat well, until pale and creamy. Crack in the egg and beat to combine.

Remove bowl from mixer and using a large, metal spoon, fold in flour and puffed millet until well blended.

Scoop out tablespoonsful of the mixture, form them into balls with your fingers and then roll them in the crushed corn flakes to coat them thoroughly.

Place cookies onto the prepared tray about 7cm (3 inches) apart and bake in oven for 15 minutes or until golden-brown.

Allow cookies to stand on tray for 2-3 minutes before sliding a spatula under each one and removing them to a wire rack to cool.

Repeat until you have used up all the cookie mixture.

Store cookies in an airtight container for up to one week.

Yields: about 30

[GF] STONE AGE HONEY CUPCAKES

For the Cupcakes:
¼ cup arrowroot
⅛ teaspoon salt
⅛ teaspoon baking soda
3 large free-range egg yolks
¼ cup HIT-friendly butter
2 tablespoons honey
1 tablespoon natural, oil-based vanilla extract

For the Frosting:
¾ cup HIT-friendly thick cream or butter
2 teaspoons maple syrup
½ teaspoon natural, oil-based vanilla extract
ground cardamom for dusting

Preheat oven to 175°C (350°F). Line a cupcake pan with 6 paper liners.

In a food processor, combine arrowroot, salt and baking soda. Pulse in egg yolks, butter, honey and vanilla.

Scoop ¼ cup into each cupcake liner. Place tray in the oven and bake for 20-24 minutes. Remove from oven and allow to cool for at least 1 hour before covering with frosting.

To make the frosting, put the cream or butter in the bowl of an electric mixer with the vanilla and maple syrup. Whip for a couple of minutes until it is fluffy.

Pipe or spread the frosting over the top of the cooled cupcakes. Sprinkle a little cardamom over the top if desired.

Store cupcakes in the fridge and take out of the fridge at least 20 minutes before eating.

Yields: 6 cupcakes

18. Jams, Jellies & Preserves

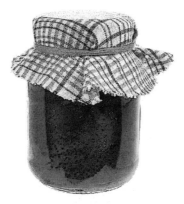

HINTS FOR MAKING JAMS AND JELLIES

When making jams and jellies, always use fruit that's in excellent condition, preferably slightly under-ripe.

Coarse-grained, white, granulated sugar is best for jam-making because the grains dissolve slowly and evenly, producing a nice, clear jam.

Use a large, heavy-bottomed saucepan or pot for jam-making. All jam-making equipment should be made of non-reactive material, such as glass, plastic, steel, earthenware, or enamel. Plastic sieves and strainers are preferred.

Testing whether jam or jelly has set properly:

You can purchase a sugar thermometer to test when jam reaches the 'setting point' (104°C/220°F), or use the following method.

Place a saucer into freezer to chill it. Take out the saucer and put a small blob of the jam onto it. Leave it for a few seconds, then tilt the saucer on an angle. If the blob stays where it is or moves slightly and sluggishly, then it has reached setting point and is ready. If it's not ready it will run, like syrupy liquid. In that case continue to boil the jam, testing every few minutes.

After the jam is ready, while it is still very hot, pour it into clean mason jars a little at a time (to stop the glass from cracking due to sudden heat), wipe off any drips and fasten on clean lids. Turn the jars upside-down for two minutes to sterilize the lids, then turn them back upright and allow them to stand cooling for a few hours. The scalding heat of the boiling hot jam will sterilize the jars.

[GF] MAKE YOUR OWN APPLE PECTIN

Jams and jellies need a compound called pectin in order to set. Some fruits are naturally high in pectin, but others have very little. You can buy liquid or powdered pectin to make your low-pectin fruit jelly or jam set to a gel, or you can make your own. Pectin should be added to the fruit before the sugar.

Apple pectin is also good for you. As mentioned, research has shown that it can obstruct the absorption of food allergens. [116] Fruit pectin has been used to treat high cholesterol, diabetes and gastroesophageal reflux disease (GERD). It binds substances in the intestine, and has also been used to help prevent colon cancer.

If you make a few liters or gallons of liquid pectin at a time, you can preserve it by freezing in batches, to use throughout the year. It is very useful not only for setting jam, but also for adding tartness to very sweet fruit jams such as mango and fig.

The only HIT-friendly jam and jelly ingredients with high pectin are apples, persimmons and quinces. The rest—rhubarb, mango, fig and melon, need additional pectin if they are going to set properly.

How to make liquid apple pectin:

To make liquid apple pectin, select under-ripe apples that are still somewhat green, hard, and sour. In general, ripe apples contain less pectin.

4 kg (9 pounds) under-ripe apples
water
rubbing alcohol, for testing (optional)

Wash the apples. You don't have to peel or core them; simply chop them into rough chunks. Pile them into a large cooking pot, then add just enough water to almost cover the apple pieces.

Bring to the boil, then cover the pot with a lid and simmer over a low heat for a long time, until the apples are fully cooked and resemble runny applesauce with skins and seeds in it. Stir the apples every twenty minutes or so while they are simmering.

When cooked, strain the hot applesauce through cheesecloth.

Note: you can line a colander with cheese-cloth for this step, or alternatively, tie a white T-shirt securely over the top of a large, clean cooking pot.

It's best not to press the applesauce to extract more pectin, because pressing it pushes some of the solids through. This makes the finished product somewhat cloudy, and also flavors it with some of the unpleasant tartness of the under-ripe apples. Ideally, leave it overnight to drain. Discard or compost the apple pulp.

The thick, clear liquid and slightly slimy that drips down from the cheesecloth is the apple pectin.

Testing the pectin's strength:

To test its strength, pour a little rubbing alcohol into a glass and then drop in a spoonful of cold (never hot) pectin. The pectin will curdle into a gelatinous blob.

Perfect: If you can scoop out this glob with a fork and it holds together in a gooey mass on the tines, then it is concentrated enough to give the perfect jell to jams and jellies.

Reasonable: If you can scoop it up with the fork, but most of it dangles loosely from the tines, then it will jell reasonably well but not perfectly.

Unacceptable: If, when you try to scoop it up the fork tines pass straight through it or you can only pick up small amounts, then the concentration is not strong enough for proper jelling. If this happens, boil it down (reducing the liquid by steam evaporation) to increase the pectin's concentration.

How much homemade pectin to use?

When making jams and jellies, make sure you use exactly the amount of sugar that the recipe calls for; otherwise you risk making a batch that will not jell. This is because jelling depends not only on the concentration of pectin, but also on the concentration of sugar.

Using less sugar won't necessarily make a 'healthier' jam—let's face it—jam by definition, is a confection full of sugar, so you may as well make it properly.

For jams: use about ¼ cup of 'perfect' homemade apple pectin per cup of low-pectin fruit. As mentioned above, pectin should be added to the fruit before the sugar. Usually the fruit-to-sugar ratio for traditional jams is 1:1, that is, 1 cup of sugar for every 1 cup of fruit.

For jellies: use 1 cup of 'perfect' homemade apple pectin per cup of low pectin fruit juice. Use ¼ cup homemade pectin if your fruit juice is already high in pectin (apples, persimmons, quinces). Measure the amount of combined pectin and juice, then add an equal amount of sugar.

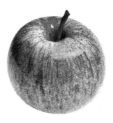

[GF] MANGO JAM

Use fruit that is firm and only just ripe. You may include a few fully ripe fruits, and perhaps one that is completely green, but never any that are over-ripe.

---

sufficient mangos to make 4 cups prepared mango
**   pulp (about 6)**
commercial¹ or homemade apple pectin
1 ¼ cups water
4 cups sugar (no less!)

---

1   Commercial pectin should be measured according to instructions on the packet.

Peel the mangos, remove the stone, and chop the pulp into thin dice. If you prefer very smooth jam, then purée the fruit. Measure 4 cups of mango flesh, then pour it into the jam-making saucepan.

Add water to the pan and set it over a medium heat. Bring the contents to the boil. Simmer gently until the fruit is reduced by about a third—it will take about 20 minutes.

Add the pectin, according to instructions on the packet.

Turn up the heat and add the sugar, 1 cup at a time, stirring constantly with a long-handled wooden spoon, till all the sugar has been blended. The jam should be continuously boiling throughout this process.

Leaves the jam on a rolling boil until the setting point is reached—about 20-30 minutes, or till a sugar thermometer reads (104°C/220°F) stirring occasionally to prevent the jam from scorching. Test whether the jam has set, using methods described above, and when it is ready, remove from heat.

Too little boiling will result in runny jam, but do not overboil, because the jam will scorch, becoming sticky and dark and losing flavor.

Allow the mango jam to stand for a few minutes. Skim off any scum with a slotted spoon. Pour the hot jam into clean, dry jars, filling them to the top.

Finish bottling the jam according to instructions above.

Spread on toast, use in baking or spoon over desserts and ice cream.

Yields: about 2 kilos (2.2 pounds).

[GF] FIG JAM

1 kg (2.2 pounds) ripe or slightly under-ripe figs, trimmed, roughly chopped
500g (17.5 ounces) sugar
1 vanilla bean, split, seeds scraped
6 cardamom pods tied in a small muslin bag
commercial[1] or homemade apple pectin

---

1   Commercial pectin should be measured according to instructions on the packet.

Place ingredients in a bowl, cover with a lid or clean dishcloth, and allow to stand overnight at room temperature.

Pour the mixture into a large saucepan, set it over a low heat and stir to dissolve sugar.

When sugar is dissolved turn heat to high, bring to the boil, then lower the heat again.

Simmer over a very low heat for about 45 minutes, , stirring regularly, until the jam becomes thick and sticky.

Gently break up figs a little with a fork. Remove vanilla bean and cardamom pouch, then cool slightly and pour into clean jars as described above, and seal. Keeps for up to 3 months.

Yields: about 2 cups

[GF] RHUBARB JAM

> **500g (17.5 ounces) trimmed red rhubarb, washed, coarsely chopped**
> **500g (17.5 ounces) sugar**
> **commercial[1] or homemade apple pectin**
> **1 teaspoon vanilla essence**
>
> ---
>
> 1   Commercial pectin should be measured according to instructions on the packet.

Combine the rhubarb, pectin, sugar, and vanilla in a large glass bowl. Cover and set aside overnight to infuse.

Pour the rhubarb mixture to your jam-making saucepan. Set over medium-high heat and bring to the boil.

Use a large slotted spoon to skim any froth from the surface. Simmer rapidly, stirring, for 25-30 minutes or until the jam jells when tested (see above).

Spoon the hot jam mixture into clean, dry jars. Finish bottling the jam according to instructions above.

Yields: about 2 ½ cups.

Variation: add 25g (1 ounce) crystallized ginger, finely chopped.

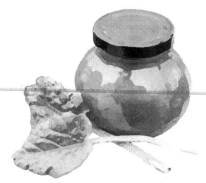

[GF] APPLE CARAMEL JAM

6 cups diced peeled apples cut into 0.3cm (⅛-inch) cubes
½ cup water
½ teaspoon HIT-friendly butter
50 g (1-¾ ounces) powdered apple pectin
3 cups sugar
2 cups packed brown sugar
½ teaspoon ground cardamom
¼ teaspoon ground allspice

In a jam-making saucepan, combine the apples, water and butter. Cook and stir over low heat until apples are tender.

Stir in pectin and bring to a rolling boil, stirring continuously. Add the sugars and spices and return to a rolling boil.

Boil for 1 minute, stirring constantly.

Remove jam pan from the heat; skim off any foam with a slotted spoon. Ladle hot mixture into clean jars, leaving ½ cm (¼ inch) headspace, and follow the jam-bottling instructions above.

Yields: 1.6 liters (3.5 pints).

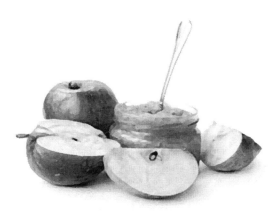

[GF] APPLE BUTTER

3 kg (6½ pounds) apples, peeled, cored and sliced[1]
1 cup white sugar
1 cup light brown sugar
1 tablespoon ground cardamom
¾ teaspoon ground allspice
¼ teaspoon salt
1 tablespoon vanilla extract

---

1   We suggest a combination of Granny Smith and some sweeter apples.

Place apples in a slow cooker. In a medium sized mixing bowl, beat the sugars, spices and salt until well combined. Sprinkle this mixture over the apples and stir gently to blend. Put the lid on and cook on low for 10 hours.

Stir in vanilla extract. With a fork, break up any large chunks of apple. Cover and cook for a further 2 hours.

Remove lid and use a stick blender to purée the apple butter until completely smooth.

If you prefer thicker apple butter, continue to cook on low with the lid slightly ajar to allow steam to escape.

When it has reached your desired consistency, turn off the cooker. Ladle hot mixture into jars, according to bottling directions above. Store in the refrigerator for up to 2 weeks, or freeze for up to 2 months.

Yield: 1.9 liters (4 pints).

[GF] PERSIMMON JELLY

> **3.6 kg (8 pounds) fresh, ripe[1], soft persimmons, washed and trimmed**
> **2 cups water**
> **7 cups white sugar**
> **commercial powdered apple pectin**
> **L-ascorbic acid powder**
>
> ——————
>
> 1   Not over-ripe!

Cut the persimmons into chunks. Remove the pits and any brown spots and mushy areas. Place them in your jam pan with the water and heat to a simmer.

Remove the softened persimmons from the heat and put them through a Foley food mill or other sieve to make a purée. If you prefer, you can whiz them in a food processor.

To keep the fruit from turning brown, sprinkle over it ¼ cup ascorbic acid powder, then stir it in.

Measure out the amount of pectin powder specified on the packet, plus about 20% more. Mix the dry pectin with about ¼ cup of sugar. Keep this separate from the rest of the sugar.

Stir the pectin into the persimmons and pour the mixture into your jam saucepan. Set on the stove over a medium to high heat and bring to the boil, stirring occasionally to prevent scorching. This should take about 5 to 10 minutes.

When the jam has reached a full boil, add the rest of the sugar cup by cup. Return it to the boil and boil rapidly for 1 minute.

Test for 'jell' using the method described above. If the jam is not yet thick enough, mix in a little more pectin (about tablespoon)and bring it to a boil again for 1 minute.

Bottle according to directions above.

[GF] MELON AND GINGER JAM

> **1 kg (2 ¼ pounds) peeled and seeded melon[1]**
> **250 g (9 ounces) preserved ginger diced[2]**
> **1 kg (2 ¼ pounds) sugar**
> **commercial[3] or homemade apple pectin**
> **1⁄4 teaspoon pepper**
>
> ---
>
> 1   Choose melons such as honeydew, cantaloupe (rock-melon) or casaba.
> 2   Or 100 g (3.5 ounces) peeled, diced fresh ginger.
> 3   Commercial pectin should be measured according to instructions on the packet.

Cut melon flesh into tiny cubes. Mix the melon, ginger and sugar in a glass, plastic, steel, earthenware, or enamel bowl and allow to stand, refrigerated, overnight.

Pour the melon, ginger and sugar into your jam saucepan and boil until the melon becomes transparent.

Add the pectin and pepper and continue to boil until the jam passes the 'jell' test, as described above.

Bottle according to instructions above.

[GF] QUINCE JELLY

> **3kg (6 pounds) ripe quinces, unpeeled**
> **approx. 1kg (2¼ pounds) white sugar[1]**
> **3 or 4 leaves of lemon scented geranium**
>   **(optional)**
>
> ---
>
> 1   Or 500g/1 pound sugar to every 600ml/1 pint of strained juice

Wash the quinces, rub off their fluff and cut into chunks, removing any blemished or rotten parts. You don't have to peel them, but do remove the cores because you are probably going to use this flesh, later, to make quince paste.

Place quinces in your jam-making saucepan and pour over enough water to just cover the fruit. Simmer until quinces are tender, which will take at least an hour.

Line a large non-reactive bowl with a few layers of cheesecloth or muslin or even an open pillowcase. Ladle all the quince pulp into the fabric, pull up the edges to form a bag and tie the mouth of the bag firmly with strong string, leaving a loop of extra string.

Hang up the bag by the loop, over the bowl. Leave it to drip overnight (or for at least 4 hours). Don't squeeze it too much, or your jelly will not turn out clear.

Measure the juice (it will probably be about 1.25 liters, i.e. 2 pints) and pour it into your jam saucepan. Measure out 500g (1 pound) of white sugar to every 600ml (1 pint) of juice.

Save the pulp in a sealed container in the refrigerator. You can make delicious quince paste with it (see recipe below).

Stir the sugar into the strained quince juice.

If you wish, you can now throw a few leaves of lemon scented geranium into the juice. Remove them later, before pouring the quince jelly into jars.

Set the jam saucepan on your stove and heat slowly, stirring occasionally to dissolve the sugar. When it is dissolved, bring to the boil rapidly. Skim any scum off the top with a slotted spoon. Boil until the jelly reaches setting point. Test for 'jell' according to instructions above.

Pot into warm, dry jars according to bottling instructions above, cover and seal.

Serve your quince jelly on crumpets, muffins or toast, or as a dessert topping. Use within 12 months.

Makes: 1.5 liters of fragrant, clear, amber-pink jelly.

[GF] QUINCE PASTE (MEMBRILLO)

> **1 quantity drained quince pulp left over from
>   quince jelly recipe
> an equal weight of white sugar
> rice bran oil spray**

Place the fruit into a food processor and blend until very smooth. Place in your jam-making saucepan with the sugar.

Cook over a low heat, stirring constantly, until the sugar dissolves. Continue to cook over the same low heat, still stirring occasionally, for 1-1½ hours, or until the quince paste has thickened and turned a deep orange color.

Preheat the oven to 50°C (120°F). Grease a 20 x 20cm (8 x 8 inch) baking tray with low sides, and line it with non-stick baking paper (parchment paper).

Pour the cooked paste into the baking tray and smooth it out evenly. Put it in the preheated oven and leave it there for one hour to speed up the setting process and help dry it out.

Remove from the oven, allow to cool and slice into manageable portions.

Store portions in sealed containers in the refrigerator.

Use membrillo as a sweet, rolled in vanilla sugar [page 220], to serve with coffee.

[GF] FIG AND APPLE PASTE

> **6 just-ripe figs, coarsely chopped
> 4 just-ripe apples peeled, cored, chopped
> ¼ cup water
> approx. 500g (17.5 ounces) white sugar**

Combine the figs, apples and water in a large saucepan over high heat. Bring to the boil. Reduce heat to low and simmer, stirring occasionally, for 30 minutes or until tender. Remove from heat and set aside for 10 minutes to cool slightly.

Transfer mixture to the bowl of a food processor and process until smooth. Weigh mixture. You will need the same weight of sugar as the purée for this recipe.

Combine the purée and sugar in a heavy-based saucepan over medium-low heat. Cook, stirring, for 10 minutes or until sugar dissolves.

Reduce heat to low and cook, stirring occasionally, for 3 hours or until mixture is very thick. Remove from heat and set aside for 30 minutes to cool slightly.

Grease the base and sides of six ½ cup (125ml) ramekins. Spoon the purée evenly among the ramekins and smooth the surface. Loosely cover with baking paper (parchment paper) and set aside for 2 days or until surface feels dry to the touch and mixture thickens.

Turn out of the ramekins and cover with plastic wrap. Store in the refrigerator

Fig and apple paste can be spread on toast, stirred into tea as a sweetener, or served as part of an appetizer. Cooks may also add it to sauces and pastry recipes to give them flavor and texture.

In addition to being used as a delicious jam, fig and apple paste typically combines well with other fruits. An entree platter might include pita chips or seeded crackers, a bowl of fig and apple paste and some HIT-friendly cream or ricotta cheese. Spreading a cracker or chip with the cream and topping it with fig and apple paste and a thin apple or pear slice usually makes a tasty pre-dinner snack.

Yields: 6 x ½ cup (125ml)

[GF] HIT-FRIENDLY PICKLES [17]

> **For Dill Pickles:**
> **1 English cucumber**
> **¼ teaspoon ascorbic acid powder**
> **½ teaspoon dill**
> **3 tablespoon salt**

Wash cucumber and cut off the ends. Use a mandoline slicer or a potato peeler to slice cucumber very thinly – the thinner you slice them, the more rapidly they will pickle.

Put all cucumber slices in a plastic container. Cover slices in salt and rub salt into the cucumber slices.

Close plastic container with a lid that seals tightly, and place in refrigerator for at least 12 hours. During this time, occasionally take it out and give it a shake.

When cucumber slices have become flexible, turn them out of the container into a colander and drain.

Run water over the cucumber slices while rubbing them continually to remove as much salt as possible. Keep rubbing and squeezing out the water. Rinse several times and taste-test to make sure the salt has decreased to your preference. Squeeze out the rest of the water and place cucumber in bowl.

Add ascorbic acid and dill. Mix well, taste, and adjust as necessary.

---

17   Adapted from 'Low Amine Recipes' by Michelle Ferris.

For Kimchee Pickles:
1 large Japanese daikon radish
½ teaspoon ascorbic acid powder
½ teaspoon onion powder
1 teaspoon garlic powder
1 green onion, thinly sliced.

Prepare the radish the same way as the cucumber, but instead of mixing the rinsed slices with dill, use the ascorbic acid powder, onion powder, garlic powder and green onion.

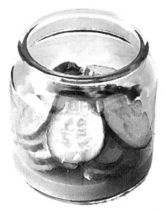

19. Desserts

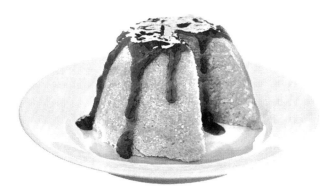

Desserts are easy to prepare on the Strictly Low Histamine Diet. Simple rice puddings can be sweetened with sugar or stevia and flavored with culinary myrtle leaves, bay leaves or cardamom. Rose extract or vanilla can flavor white blancmange. Stewed fruits can be topped with a rolled oats/flour/sugar/butter crumble topping and served with a dollop of HIT-friendly cream. Bread and butter pudding can be laced with fig jam.

Here are some more ideas.

SWEET BLACK RICE DESSERTS

Sticky rice is popular in Vietnam, Japan, Indonesia and other Asian countries. The black-hued variety is usually boiled, sweetened and served as a dessert. When cooked, the rice acquires a viscous texture and turns a deep purplish colour, which adds a delightful vibrancy to dishes.

Black glutinous rice is a short-grained variety of black rice that contains no gluten. It is also referred to as 'sticky' or 'sweet' black rice. According to a 2010 report from the American Chemical Society, black rice may have even more health benefits than brown rice. Black rice bran contains high levels of anthocyanins, water soluble antioxidants that are found in blue and purple fruits. The rice is high in fiber, vitamins and minerals, and possesses anti-inflammatory properties that reduce allergy, asthma and other disease symptoms.

You can buy black glutinous rice, pandan leaves, palm sugar and lemongrass from Asian grocery stores or online.

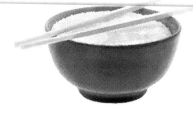

[GF] SWEET BLACK RICE PUDDING WITH PANDAN

> 1½ cups black glutinous rice
> 6 cups water
> 1 pandan or screw-pine leaf, tied in a knot[1]
> ½ - ¾ cup (100 - 150g) (3 ½ - 5 ounces) palm
>   sugar, chopped
> 400ml (14 fluid ounces) HIT-friendly milk
> ¼ teaspoon salt
>
> ---
>
> 1   Pandan leaves can be bought at your local Asian food
> store or online.

Wash the rice thoroughly and soak it in cold water several hours or overnight.

Drain rice and combine with the water in a large saucepan. Bring to a boil stirring occasionally.

Reduce heat to a simmer. Add pandan leaf and cook, partially covered, about 30 minutes or until rice is very tender stirring occasionally. Rice should still be fairly wet.

Add sugar and stir until it dissolves into the rice. Remove pandan leaf. Rice may be eaten warm, but is preferable at room temperature or cold.

Before serving, combine milk and salt in a medium jug; stir to dissolve salt.

Serve rice drizzled with salted milk.

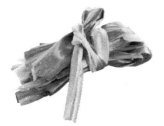

[GF] BLACK STICKY RICE WITH MANGOS AND SWEET CARDAMOM SAUCE

> **2 cups black sticky rice**
> **4 cups water**
> **1 fresh pandan leaf (optional)[1]**
>
> **Sweet cardamom sauce:**
> **1 cup shaved palm sugar or brown sugar**
> **2½ cups thick, heavy HIT-friendly cream**
> **½ teaspoon ground cardamom**
> **½ teaspoon salt**
>
> **Topping:**
> **2 ripe mangos peeled, stone removed and sliced**
> **2 teaspoons toasted black cumin seeds**
> _____
> 1   If you cannot find pandan leaf, try substituting natural, oil-based vanilla extract plus green food coloring made from basil—"[GF] Green Food Dyes" on page 130. It will give a different flavor, however. Pandan has a unique taste.

Rinse the black rice under running water for a few minutes then place in a saucepan with the water and the pandan leaf tied in a knot.

Bring rice slowly to the boil then reduce the heat and simmer slowly until all the water is absorbed. This will take about 30 minutes.

Meanwhile, to make the cardamom sauce heat the palm sugar, cardamom, milk and salt together in a saucepan over medium heat for about 5 minutes, stirring constantly, until the sugar is dissolved. Set aside.

When the rice is cooked remove the saucepan from the heat and pour half of the cardamom sauce into the rice. Stir, then cover with foil and allow to stand so that the rice can absorb the sauce and the mixture can thicken. This will take about 10-15 minutes.

To serve, place small portions of the sticky rice on individual plates, drizzle over the remaining sauce and top with slices of mango and a sprinkling of toasted black cumin seeds.

[GF] SWEET BLACK RICE PUDDING WITH LEMONGRASS

375g (13 ounces) black glutinous rice
2 stalks lemon grass, white section only, bruised
2 vanilla beans, split
400ml (14 fluid ounces) HIT-friendly milk
1 cup oat milk [page 94]
1 cup water
3/4 cup finely chopped palm sugar
1 1/2 tablespoons HIT-friendly butter
4 figs cut into thick wedges, or 1 ripe mango, sliced.
2 tablespoons HIT-friendly cream, to garnish

Place the rice in a large bowl and cover with cold water. Cover with plastic wrap and set aside overnight to soak.

Drain rice. Rinse under cold running water. Drain well. Combine the rice, lemon grass, vanilla beans, milk, oat milk, water and ½ cup palm sugar in a large saucepan over low heat. Bring to a simmer. Cook, stirring occasionally, for 1 ½ hours or until liquid is almost absorbed and rice is tender and creamy.

Heat the butter in a medium frying pan over medium heat until foaming but not smoking. Add the figs and cook for 2-3 minutes or until golden. Sprinkle over the remaining sugar and cook, stirring, for 2 minutes or until sugar dissolves and fig caramelizes.

Remove and discard lemon grass and vanilla beans from rice. Spoon the rice evenly among serving bowls. Top with figs or mango and drizzle with any pan juices and extra cream. Serve immediately.

[GF] TOFFEE MELON BALLS WITH GINGER CREAM

> 1 cup HIT-friendly cream mixed with ½ teaspoon
>   pure vanilla or HIT-friendly vanilla substitute
> 1 tablespoon finely chopped glacé ginger
> 700g (25 ounces) small cantaloupe (rockmelon),
>   seeded
> 700g (25 ounces) small honeydew melon, seeded
> ½ cup caster sugar
> sprigs of mint, to garnish (optional)

Combine vanilla, cream and ginger in a bowl.

Using a melon baller (or a teaspoon if you don't have one), scoop spheres of colored flesh from rockmelon and honeydew melon.

Place them on a large plate lined with paper towel. Cover with paper towel and pat dry.

Combine caster sugar and ¼ cup hot water in a small heavy-based saucepan over low heat. Cook, stirring, for 4 minutes or until sugar is dissolved.

Increase heat to high. Bring to the boil. Boil, without stirring, for 8 minutes or until mixture turns golden.

Set aside for 30 seconds for bubbles to subside.

Arrange melon balls in a large serving bowl. Drizzle over toffee. Stand at room temperature for 5 minutes or until toffee is set and cooled. Serve immediately with ginger cream and garnish with fresh mint if desired.

Serves: 4

[GF] TRAFFIC LIGHT MELONS IN CARDAMOM SYRUP

> 1 x 270ml (9 fluid ounces) HIT-friendly milk
> ½ teaspoon ground cardamom
> 75g (5 tablespoons) caster sugar
> 6 kaffir lime leaves, crushed
> 1 x 10cm (4 inch) piece—pale section only—fresh
>   lemon grass, halved lengthways
> ¼ watermelon, peeled, cut into 3cm (1 inch) cubes
> ¼ rockmelon, peeled, cut into 3cm (1 inch) cubes
> ¼ honeydew melon, peeled, cut into 3cm (1 inch)
>   cubes (or scooped out in balls)

Combine cardamom, milk, sugar, kaffir lime leaves and lemon grass in a saucepan over medium heat.

Bring to boil. Reduce heat and simmer, uncovered, for 8-10 minutes or until reduced to a syrup consistency.

Set aside for 10 minutes to cool. Strain and discard the lemon grass and lime leaves.

Arrange watermelon, rockmelon and honeydew melon in bowls and drizzle with cardamom syrup.

Serves: 4

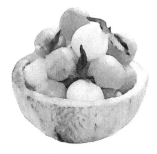

[GF] JEWELED MELON FRUIT SALAD

⅓ cup honey
½ teaspoon natural vanilla bean paste
1.2kg (2 ½ pounds) cantaloupe (rockmelon), cut
    into 5cm (2 inch) pieces
1kg (2 ¼ pounds) honeydew melon, cut into 5cm
    (2 inch) pieces
800g (28 ounces) seedless watermelon, cut into
    5cm (2 inch) pieces

Place honey, vanilla and ¼ cup cold water in a saucepan over medium heat. Bring to the boil. Reduce heat to medium-low. Simmer for 5 minutes or until mixture thickens slightly. Set aside to cool.

Combine rockmelon, honeydew and watermelon in a bowl. Drizzle with honey mixture. Serve.

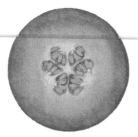

[GF] CARDAMOM ICE-CREAM WITH RHUBARB AND MELON FRUIT SALAD

375ml (13 fluid ounces) HIT-friendly milk
1/3 cup whipped HIT-friendly cream
⅓ teaspoon ground cardamom
2 tablespoons caster sugar
1 1/2 teaspoons powdered agar agar
1/2 small cantaloupe (rockmelon), seeded, peeled,
    thinly sliced
1/2 small honeydew melon, seeded, peeled, thinly
    sliced
1/2 cup red rhubarb, stewed with 2 tablespoons
    sugar and puréed

Place milk, cream, cardamom and sugar in a small saucepan over medium-low heat. Heat, stirring occasionally, for 5 to 6 minutes or until almost simmering (don't boil). Remove from heat and immediately sprinkle agar agar powder over it. Whisk until agar dissolves. Set aside for 10 minutes to cool.

Pour cream mixture into a 6cm-deep, 11cm x 21cm (base) loaf pan. If you don't have a loaf pan, you can use a 2 liter-capacity freezer container.

Cover surface with plastic wrap, then foil. Freeze for 2 hours or until frozen around edge of pan. Transfer to a bowl. Using an electric mixer, beat until mixture is light and fluffy and doubled in size. Return to pan. Cover surface with plastic wrap, then foil. Repeat freezing and beating process. Freeze for 6 hours or overnight.

Remove ice-cream from freezer. Stand for 5 minutes to soften slightly. Meanwhile, combine rockmelon, honeydew melon and puréed cooked rhubarb in a large bowl. Scoop ice-cream and serve with rhubarb and melon salad.

Serves: 6

JAMMY PIKELETS WITH CARDAMOM CREAM

For Pikelets:
1 cup self-raising flour with permitted
    ingredients[1]
⅓ cup caster sugar
pinch of bicarbonate of soda
¾ cup oat milk
1 free-range egg
melted HIT-friendly butter, to grease
½ cup fig or persimmon jam

For Cardamom Cream:
500g (1 pound) whipped light HIT-friendly cream
    ["Cream Substitutes" on page 106]
¼ cup caster sugar
2 tablespoons oat milk
½ teaspoon ground cardamom

---

1   To make self-raising flour, add 2 teaspoons of baking powder and ½ teaspoon salt to a cup of all-purpose flour.

Sift the flour, sugar and bicarbonate of soda into a medium sized mixing bowl and make a well in the center.

Whisk together milk and egg in a jug. Use a wooden spoon to gradually stir milk mixture into dry ingredients, beating gently until smooth.

Brush a non-stick frypan lightly with melted butter to grease it, and place over medium-low heat. To make four pikelets, pour four dessertspoonsful of batter into pan from the tip of the spoon, each about 4cm (1 ½ inches) apart. Cook for 1-2 minutes or until golden underneath and bubbles appear on surface.

Turn pikelets over and cook other side for 30 seconds or until golden underneath. Transfer to a wire rack to cool.

Repeat with remaining batter, greasing pan lightly with melted HIT-friendly butter before cooking each batch.

To make Cardamom Cream, place HIT-friendly cream, sugar, milk and cardamom in a mixing bowl. Use an electric beater to whisk until well combined and fluffy.

To serve, top each pikelet with one teaspoon of jam and one tablespoon of Cardamom Cream.

Yield: about 28 pikelets

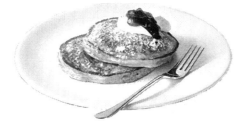

STEAMED FIG PUDDINGS EN CREUSE

½ cup brown sugar, firmly packed
80g (3 ounces) HIT-friendly butter, at room
    temperature
¾ teaspoon ground cardamom
¾ teaspoon ground allspice
1 teaspoon natural, oil-based vanilla essence
2 free-range egg yolks, lightly whisked
100g (3 ½ ounces) HIT-friendly sour
    cream [page 105]
1 cup self-raising flour with permitted
    ingredients[1], sifted
150g (5 ounces) fresh figs, finely chopped
melted butter, for greasing
To serve: whipped HIT-friendly cream flavored
    with pure vanilla or HIT-friendly vanilla sub-
    stitute, or "Cardamom Ice-cream"

---

1   To make self-raising flour, add 2 teaspoons of baking
powder and ½ teaspoon salt to a cup of all-purpose flour.

Preheat oven to 200°C (400°F). Brush six 250ml (1 cup) ovenproof dishes, teacups or flat-based ramekins with the melted butter to grease.

Using the top of a dish or ramekin as a guide, cut six discs of non-stick baking paper (parchment paper) and set aside. Line the bases with extra non-stick baking paper.

Use electric beaters to beat the sugar, butter, spice and vanilla essence in a medium bowl until pale and creamy. Add the egg yolks one at a time, beating after each addition until well combined (the mixture will look slightly curdled).

Add the sour cream, flour and figs to the butter mixture and use a wooden spoon or spatula to fold in until well combined.

Divide the mixture among the ramekins and use the back of the spoon to smooth the surface of each. Top each with a disc of baking paper, trimming the discs if necessary so they sit on top of the pudding mixture.

Place the ramekins in a roasting pan. Add enough boiling water to the pan to reach halfway up their sides.

Bake in preheated oven for 30 minutes or until a skewer inserted in the center of the puddings comes out clean.

Run a round-bladed knife around the edge of each pudding to loosen. Carefully turn onto serving plates and serve immediately, drizzled with HIT-friendly cream or accompanied by HIT-friendly ice-cream.

Serves: 6

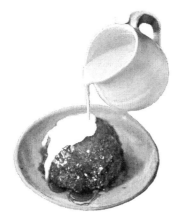

APPLE AND RHUBARB CRUMBLE

**1 bunch (425g or 15 ounces) rhubarb, cut into
    2cm (1 inch) pieces
3 Granny Smith apples, peeled, cored and sliced
2 tablespoons caster sugar
1/2 tablespoon amchoor [page 114]
1/4 cup green mango juice
3/4 cup plain all purpose flour with permitted
    ingredients1, sifted
3/4 cup rolled oats
100g HIT-friendly butter, chilled, cubed
1/4 cup brown sugar
1/2 cup pearl barley
1 cup water
2 teaspoons rice bran oil**

---

1   To make self-raising flour, add 2 teaspoons of baking
powder and ½ teaspoon salt to a cup of all-purpose flour.

Toasted Pearl Barley:

Simmer the barley in a cup of water, for 30 to 45 minutes or until tender. You may need to top up the water occasionally. Drain.

Heat the rice bran oil in a small frypan and toast the cooked barley grains until brown. Set aside. [18]

Filling and Topping:

Preheat oven to 180°C (350°F). Place rhubarb, apple, sugar, amchoor and juice into a rectangular ovenproof dish 26cx 16cm (10 x 6 inches). Stir until well-blended.

Combine flour and rolled oats in a large bowl. Add butter. Using your fingertips, rub butter into flour and oat mixture. Stir

---

18   Note: it is useful to keep on hand a stock of cooked and toasted barley grains for use in cooking. They have a mild, nutty flavor and are very nutritious—a good substitute for nuts. Store in sealed bags in the freezer.

in sugar and toasted barley. Sprinkle over rhubarb and apple mixture.

Bake for 45 minutes or until crumble is golden brown. Serve immediately, with whipped HIT-friendly cream or ice cream.

Serves: 4

ROSY RHUBARB CONFECTION

350g (12 ounces) trimmed red rhubarb, washed
    and chopped
¼ cup (55g or 2 ounces) caster sugar
2 tablespoons water
1 teaspoon rosewater
400g (14 ounces) whipped HIT-friendly cream
1 teaspoon pure vanilla or HIT-friendly vanilla
    substitute
⅓ cup caramelized pearl barley [page 284]

Place rhubarb in a saucepan and sprinkle sugar and water over. Cover and cook over medium heat for 5 minutes. Turn off heat and allow to stand for further 3 minutes. Stir through rosewater. Cool.

Meanwhile, whip the vanilla (or HIT-friendly substitute) into the cream.

Divide rhubarb between 4 wide, stemmed glasses. Top with cream and sprinkle with caramelized pearl barley.

Serve immediately.

[GF] MOIST AND JUICY RED RHUBARB PIE

3 cups plain (all-purpose) gluten free flour with
   permitted ingredients [page 194]
1 ½ cups brown sugar
1 cup HIT-friendly butter, softened
4 free-range egg yolks
another ¼ cup plain (all-purpose) gluten free
   flour with permitted ingredients [page 194]
1 ½ cups white sugar
1 cup oat milk [page 94]
½ teaspoon salt
4 cups chopped red rhubarb

Preheat oven to 175°C (350°F)

Mix 3 cups flour and brown sugar in a large bowl. Cut in softened butter with a knife or pastry blender until mixture resembles coarse crumbs.

Reserve 1 ½ cups of this crumbly flour mixture and pat the remainder into the bottom of a 22 x 33cm (9x13 inch) oven-proof pan to form the lower crust of the pie.

Bake in preheated oven until crust is lightly browned. It should take about 15 minutes.

Meanwhile, beat egg yolks in a large bowl, then add ¼ cup flour, white sugar, oat milk, and salt into egg yolks, beating until smooth.

Sprinkle chopped rhubarb over baked crust. Pour egg mixture over rhubarb; top with reserved crumbly flour mixture.

Bake in preheated oven until egg topping is set and lightly browned; 40 to 45 minutes.

Serves: 4

[GF] VANILLA BAKED FIGS

> **1 cup vanilla sugar {page 220}**
> **6 fresh figs (ripe but not over-ripe)**
> **rice bran oil spray, to grease**

Preheat oven to 220°C (430°F).

Generously grease a high-sided gratin or baking dish (the figs should fit snugly inside).

Place the sugar in a bowl. Wash figs carefully and while still damp, roll in the sugar to coat well. Roll them a second time if necessary.

Place any remaining sugar and 2 tablespoons cold water in the base of the dish. Add the figs and bake for 10 minutes until the sugar mixture forms a rich sauce (checking occasionally to ensure figs are not burning).

Set aside to cool slightly, then refrigerate for 30 minutes to chill. Serve the baked figs drizzled with a little sauce.

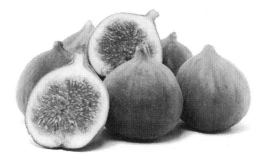

[GF] BAKED RHUBARB AND APPLE WITH SWEET DUKKAH

1 ½ cups (135g or 4 ½ ounces) rolled oats
1 ½ cups (375ml or 12 fluid ounces) fresh mango
    juice
1 Granny Smith apple, peeled, roughly grated
½ cup (120g or 4 ounces) unsweetened
    HIT-friendly cream, plus extra to serve
honey, to drizzle
sweet dukkah (see below), to serve

Baked rhubarb:
1 bunch rhubarb, stems cut into 3cm lengths
½ firmly packed cup (100g or 3 ½ ounces) brown
    sugar
½ teaspoon ground cardamom

For the sweet dukkah:
⅓ cup (4 tablespoons) black cumin seeds
2 tablespoons linseeds
⅔ cup toasted rolled oats
¼ cup (40g or 1 ½ ounces) cooked pearl barley
1 teaspoon ground allspice
1 teaspoon ground cardamom
1 teaspoon ground ginger
olive oil, to drizzle
1 tablespoon honey

Place the oats and mango juice in a bowl and stir to combine. Cover and leave to soak in the fridge overnight.

For the sweet dukkah, Preheat the oven to 200°C (400°F). Line a baking tray with baking paper (parchment paper).

Combine seeds, oats, pearl barley and spices, and spread on the tray. Drizzle with a little olive oil and toast in the oven for 4 minutes.

Remove from oven. Add honey and stir to combine. Return to oven and toast for a further 5-7 minutes until golden. Allow to cool completely, then pulse in a food processor until roughly chopped. Set aside.

For the baked rhubarb, preheat the oven to 190°C (380°F). Put the rhubarb, ½ cup brown sugar and cardamom into a baking dish and combine them. Cover with foil and bake for 10 minutes until rhubarb is softened but maintains its shape.

When ready to serve, in a mixing bowl combine the apple and cream with the mango-soaked oats and combine well.

To serve, place a few dollops of oat mixture in serving bowls or tall glasses, followed by a layer of rhubarb and topped with extra cream and a drizzle of honey. Sprinkle with sweet dukkah.

Serves: 4

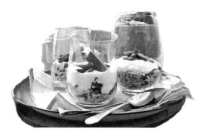

[GF] AUTUMN QUINCE TART

> **2 cups plain (all-purpose) flour with permitted ingredients**
> **1 tablespoon baking powder**
> **½ teaspoon salt**
> **½ cup sugar**
> **125g (4 ounces) HIT-friendly butter, chilled**
> **1 teaspoon natural, oil-based vanilla extract**
> **1 free-range egg**
> **1 free-range egg yolk**
> **2 tablespoons oat milk [page 94]**
> **1 cup quince paste, store-bought or homemade ["[GF] Quince Paste (Membrillo)" on page 242]**
> **¼ cup mango jam (optional) [page 234]**
> **¼ cup rhubarb jam (optional) [page 236]**
> **rice bran oil spray, to grease**

Mix the dry ingredients (flour, salt, baking powder, and sugar) together in a medium bowl.

Cut the butter into pieces, and mix butter into dry ingredients using a pastry cutter or 2 knives, until well blended.

Stir egg, egg yolk and oat milk together and add to flour mixture, blending gently with a fork until dough comes together. Knead a couple of times to just barely mix the dough, which should not be too crumbly nor too wet. If needed, add an extra tablespoon or so of flour or milk.

Wrap dough in plastic wrap and chill for at least 30 minutes.

Add quince paste (and mango jam and rhubarb jam, if using) to a small saucepan, with 1-2 tablespoons of water. Heat over low heat, stirring frequently, until mixture has melted enough to be smooth and have a spreadable consistency. Add a little more water if necessary. Remove from heat and let cool slightly.

Preheat oven to 180°C (350°F). Grease a 22 cm (9 inch) diameter round tart pan with a removable base.

Roll out about ¾ of the dough on a floured surface in a circle large enough to line the bottom and sides of the tart pan. Place the dough in the pan. Spread the filling evenly over the dough.

Roll the remaining dough into a circle, and cut thin strips of dough, using them to make a lattice pattern over the top of the tart.

Brush the tart lightly with an egg wash (1 egg thinned with 1 tablespoon water), and bake until golden brown (about 30 minutes).

At the end of the cooking time when the cake is taken out of the oven, it should be painted all over with honey (while it's hot, the honey will melt) and it should be sprinkled with icing sugar (powdered sugar) or finely chopped rolled oats (old-fashioned oats).

Serve warm or at room temperature.

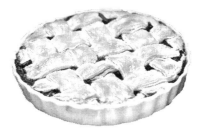

[GF] APPLE AND FIG TART

> **2 cups (300g or 10 ½ ounces) plain (all-purpose) gluten free flour with permitted ingredients [page 194]**
> **¼ cup (60g or 2 ounces) caster sugar**
> **150g (5 ounces) butter, chopped**
> **2 tablespoons iced water**
> **3 Granny Smith apples, peeled, cores removed**
> **2 tablespoons caster sugar, extra**
> **2 figs, cut into quarters**
> **2 tablespoons chopped rolled oats (old-fashioned oats)**
> **2 - 3 extra figs, sliced, to decorate**
> **3 teaspoons honey, plus extra to drizzle**
> **HIT-friendly whipped cream, to serve**

Process flour, caster sugar and butter until coarse crumbs form. Add water. Process just until mixture starts to come together. Wrap the dough in plastic. Refrigerate for 30 minutes.

Preheat oven to 180°C (350°F). Roll dough out on non-stick baking paper (parchment paper) or on a lightly floured surface until 5mm thick.

Use pastry to line a 20cm (8 inch) fluted flan tin with a removable base. Trim the edge and prick base with a fork. Line with non-stick baking paper and fill with rice or baking beans. Bake for 10 minutes.

Remove paper and rice. Bake for another 8 minutes. If base puffs up slightly, push down very gently with the end of a wooden spoon.

Thinly slice apples and toss with the extra caster sugar. Cut each fig quarter lengthways into three thin wedges.

Sprinkle chopped rolled oats over the pastry base. Arrange the apple in a spiral to make two layers of apple. Reserve the smaller pieces to fill the space in the middle.

Arrange figs evenly over the top layer by tucking them between the apples. Place extra fig slices in the middle.

Drizzle apples and figs with the honey. Bake for 30 minutes. Drizzle with extra honey and brush over the fruit. Set aside to cool slightly. Serve with cream.

Serves: 12

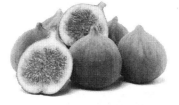

[GF] MANGO TART

Crust:
1 ¼ cups plain (all-purpose) gluten free flour with permitted ingredients [page 194]
¼ cup icing sugar (confectioners' sugar or powdered sugar)
¼ teaspoon salt
8 tablespoons cold HIT-friendly butter, cut up
3 tablespoons (or more, as needed) ice water

Tangy Pastry Cream:
1 cup oat milk [page 94]
3 large free-range egg yolks
⅓ cup white sugar
2 tablespoons cornflour (cornstarch)
2 tablespoons HIT-friendly butter
1 teaspoon amchoor [page 114]

Fruit Topping:
2 mangos, peeled and thinly sliced
Optional: a handful of thin "[GF] Candied Rhubarb Ribbons" on page 288.

Prepare crust: In food processor with knife blade attached, combine flour, confectioners' sugar, and salt; pulse until blended. Add butter and pulse until mixture resembles coarse meal.

Add ice water, 1 tablespoon at a time, pulsing until moist clumps form. Gather dough into ball; flatten into disk. Wrap disk in plastic wrap and refrigerate until firm enough to roll, about 1 hour. (If chilled overnight, let dough stand 30 minutes at room temperature before rolling.)

Preheat oven to 200°C (400°F). On lightly floured surface, with floured rolling pin, roll disk into 11-inch round.

Transfer dough round to 22 x 2.5cm (9 x 1 inch) round tart pan with removable base.

Press dough onto bottom and up sides of pan. Trim dough level with rim of pan; discard trimmings. For a bakery perfect-looking crust, the easiest and neatest way to trim dough even with the rim of a tart pan is to run a rolling pin across the top of the pan so that the metal edge cuts through the dough.

Refrigerate or freeze tart shell 10 to 15 minutes to firm dough slightly before baking.

Line tart shell with foil and fill with pie weights or dry beans. Bake 20 minutes. Remove foil and weights, and bake about 15 minutes longer or until golden. (Cover rim of tart with foil if browning too quickly.) If center of crust puffs up during baking, gently press down with back of spoon. Cool in pan on wire rack, about 30 minutes.

Meanwhile, prepare Tangy Pastry Cream. In 2-quart saucepan, heat milk to simmering on medium. In small bowl, whisk yolks and granulated sugar until blended. Mix in cornstarch until smooth. While constantly beating with wire whisk, gradually pour about half of simmering milk into egg-yolk mixture.

Pour egg-yolk mixture into remaining milk in saucepan and cook, whisking constantly to prevent lumping, until mixture boils and thickens, about 1 minute. Boil 1 minute, stirring. Remove saucepan from heat; stir in butter and amchoor.

Transfer pastry cream to small bowl; cover surface directly with plastic wrap to prevent skin from forming, and refrigerate until cold, at least 1 hour.

Spoon pastry cream into baked tart shell and spread evenly. Arrange mango slices on top; place curls of candied rhubarb ribbons in center. Remove tart from side of pan. Place tart, still on pan base, on serving plate. If not serving tart right away, cover and refrigerate up to 2 hours.

20. Snacks to Go

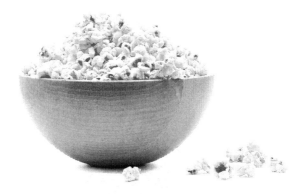

It's useful to carry low-histamine snacks with you, so that you are not tempted to eat risky foods if you feel hungry and there's nothing else available.

HIT-friendly cookies and muesli bars; fresh or candied HIT-friendly fruits such as apples, mangos and figs; sweet muffins or cupcakes; caramelized barley or popcorn; or a fruit smoothie in a thermos can provide a sweet snack. Or try a caramel flavoured milkshake!

Crispy noodles, savory muffins, popcorn, crackers and bread-sticks offer a savory way to assuage hunger.

HIT-friendly, fiber-rich grain cereals can be eaten dry from a baggie (check the ingredients on the packet).

If refrigeration is available, for example at your workplace, bring along the yolks of some hard-boiled eggs, or a dip ["[GF] Pink Party Dip" on page 154] to eat with rice crackers.

Sandwiches can be made using wheat-free, soy-free, yeast-free breads spread with HIT-friendly butter. Suggested fillings include salads, chopped hard-boiled egg yolks mixed with HIT-friendly mayonnaise, or for a sweet treat, mango jam or fig jam.

[GF] CRISPY RICE NOODLES

> **1 package thin dried rice noodles, from your supermarket Asian section**
> **¾ to 1 cup rice bran oil for frying**
> **pinch salt**

Separate rice noodles by pulling apart the various sections into manageable amounts. Using scissors, cut the noodles into 4-5 inch lengths.

Now place oil in a wok or small to medium frying pan (the smaller the pan, the less oil you will have to use). Heat oil over medium-high heat for a minimum of 1 minute.

The key to making crispy noodles is having the oil hot enough. Be sure to test it before dunking in the noodles, or you'll waste them. To test, take a few longer noodle pieces in your hand and dunk in just the ends. When the oil is hot enough, the submerged parts will 'bloom' within seconds into puffy, crispy noodles. If this doesn't happen, remove the submerged parts and cut them off. Wait a little longer for your oil to heat up, then try again.

Now gently drop handfuls of noodles in the hot oil. Have a utensil at the ready to quickly flip them once, then remove. The actual cooking time is only a few seconds. Set puffed noodles to drain on paper towels and shake over a little salt.

Continue frying the rest of the noodles, reducing heat as you do so to medium (or a fraction higher).

Use your crispy noodles as a topping for stir-fries, salad wraps, soups, salads, and other Asian dishes. Crispy noodles also make a great snack.

Storage: Crispy noodles are best eaten on the day they are made, but you can store them in tightly sealed plastic containers overnight or longer. How long they will stay crispy depends largely on the climate and level of humidity where you live.

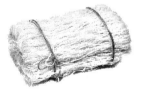

[GF] PLAIN POPCORN

> **3 tablespoons rice bran oil**
> **⅓ cup good quality popcorn kernels**
> **2 tablespoons or more (to taste) HIT-friendly butter**
> **salt to taste**

Heat the oil in a 3 liter (3 quart) saucepan on medium high heat.

Put 3 or 4 popcorn kernels into the oil and cover the pan with a well-fitted lid.

When the kernels pop, add the rest of the ⅓ cup of popcorn kernels in an even layer.

Note: If you add the salt to the oil in the pan before putting in the kernels, then when the popcorn pops, the salt will be well distributed throughout.

Cover with lid, remove from heat and count 30 seconds. This method first heats the oil to the right temperature, then waiting 30 seconds brings all of the other kernels to a near-popping temperature so that when they are put back on the heat, they all pop at about the same time.

Return the pan to the heat. The popcorn should begin popping soon, and all at once. Once the popping starts in earnest, gently shake the pan by moving it back and forth over the burner.

Try to keep the lid slightly ajar to let the steam from the popcorn release (the popcorn will be drier and crisper). Once the popping slows to several seconds between pops, remove the pan from the heat, remove the lid, and dump the popcorn immediately into a wide bowl.

Place the butter in the now empty, but hot pan to let it melt. Pour melted butter over popcorn and add salt to taste.

Topping variation: black cumin seeds.

Yield: Makes about 2 liters (2 quarts).

TWICE-BAKED BREADFINGERS

**2 cups self-raising flour with permitted
  ingredients[1]**
**1 ½ cups plain (all-purpose) flour with permitted
  ingredients**
½ tablespoon baking powder
½ teaspoon salt
⅔ cup HIT-friendly butter
⅔ cup white sugar
1 free-range egg
¾ cup buttermilk
1 teaspoon bicarb soda (baking soda)
black cumin seeds, to sprinkle
rice bran oil spray

1   To make self-raising flour, add 2 teaspoons of baking
powder and ½ teaspoon salt to a cup of all-purpose flour.

Pre-heat oven to 160°C (320°F).Spray the interior of a loaf tin by spraying it well with rice bran oil. Line the base with baking paper (parchment paper).

Melt the butter in a saucepan oven moderate heat and add sugar.

Sift the self-raising flour, plain flour, baking powder and salt.

Add the bicarb soda to the buttermilk. Add the butter, buttermilk and egg to the flour mixture and combine well. The texture should be very dry.

Place the mixture in the bread tin and sprinkle with seeds, and gently press the seeds into the mixture.

Bake for about an hour, or until a metal skewer, when inserted, comes out clean.

Remove from the oven, turn out of loaf tin and allow to dry on a drying rack.

Gently cut into fingers. Place the fingers on a baking tray sprayed with rice bran oil and place in the oven on 120°C (250°F) for about 8 hours or overnight. Serve with coffee or tea.

ITALIAN GRISSINI TWISTS

> **2 cups plain (all-purpose) flour with permitted ingredients**
> **½ teaspoon baking powder**
> **1 ½ teaspoons salt, plus more for sprinkling**
> **3 tablespoons cold HIT-friendly butter, unsalted, cut into 1.5cm (½-inch) pieces**
> **½ cup plus 1 tablespoon ice water**
> **extra-virgin olive oil, for brushing**

Preheat the oven to 190°C (375°F). In a food processor, pulse the flour with the baking powder and 1 ½ teaspoons of salt. Add the butter and pulse until the mixture resembles small peas. With the machine on, add the ice water and process just until the dough comes together.

Transfer the dough to a lightly floured work surface and pat it into a 2.5 cm (1 inch) thick rectangle. Roll out the dough to a 25 x 30 cm (10 x 12 inch) rectangle about 0.5cm (¼ inch) thick. Cut the dough crosswise into 0.5cm (¼-inch) thick strips.

Gently roll each strip into a 35 cm (14inches) long stick. (The dough can actually be rolled out to any length you prefer.)

Brush 1 stick with water and twist it with another stick, pressing at the top and the bottom.

Arrange the twists on a baking sheet. Repeat with the remaining sticks.

Brush the twists with olive oil and sprinkle with salt. Bake for about 25 minutes, until golden. Let cool before serving.

Variation: Add 2 tablespoons of black cumin seeds to the flour.

Yield: Makes about 18 breadsticks

[GF] BROWN RICE CRACKERS

> **1 cup cooked brown rice**
> **1.5 cups brown rice flour**
> **1 teaspoon salt**
> **a dash of olive oil**
> **⅓ cup hemp seeds**
> **water**
> **black cumin seeds (optional)**

Preheat oven to 190°C (375°F).

Mix cooked rice in a bowl with the brown rice flour.

Add the salt, olive oil, hemp seeds and a few drops of water and mix until dough has formed, adding more water if necessary.

Form dough into small balls and press onto an oiled baking tray, rolling out crackers out very thinly.

Bake for about 15 minutes, or until they've browned.

Remove from tray and cool on a wire rack. When cool, store in an airtight container to keep them crisp and fresh.

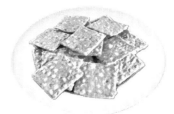

[GF] DRIED MANGO SLICES

Dried mango is truly delicious. The drying process concentrates the mango flavor and lends a chewy texture.

If you own a food dehydrator, it's best to use that. Peel and slice the mango, distribute it on the drying racks without the slices touching, and follow the instructions for your machine.

If you do not own a food dehydrator, here's how to do it.

2 ripe mangos

Preheat oven to 85°C (185°F), or as low as your oven will go. Line a baking tray with baking paper (parchment paper).

Wash mangos and use a vegetable peeler to remove the skin.

Cut mangos into thin slices and place them on the lined tray.

Put the mango slices in the oven and allow to dry for two to three hours, flipping them over every 30 minutes or until they're dry. Avoid drying for too long, or you'll end up with carboardy mango crisps!

Store in an airtight container. They are preservative-free, so use them within a few days or else freeze them.

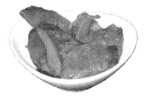

[GF] SALTED BROWN-SUGAR POPCORN

Yield: 6 servings

> **6 cups popped popcorn**
> **¾ cup dark brown sugar**
> **¼ cup water**
> **1 tablespoon HIT-friendly butter**
> **1 teaspoon natural, oil-based, alcohol-free vanilla extract**
> **1 tablespoon HIT-friendly milk of your choice (e.g. oat, brown rice)**
> **1 tsp sea salt (or more, according to your taste)**

Pour the popcorn into a heatproof bowl.

Place brown sugar, water, butter and vanilla extract into a small saucepan and stir until combined.

Put the saucepan on the stovetop and bring to a boil without stirring.

Pour in the milk and cook until the mixture thickens. This should take about five minutes.

Remove saucepan from heat, add salt and stir it in, then pour the mixture over the popped popcorn.

Stir the popcorn to make sure it is coated all over with the brown sugar mixture, then tip it out onto a baking sheet.

Spread out the popcorn evenly and let it cool at room temperature for two to three hours before eating.

[GF] CANDIED SWEET POTATOES

> **100g (2 pounds) sweet potatoes or yams,**
> **preferably with yellow or orange flesh**
> **⅓ cup tightly packed brown sugar**
> **3 tablespoons HIT-friendly butter**
> **3 tablespoons water**
> **½ teaspoon salt**

Scrub sweet potatoes, but do not peel. Place sweet potatoes in 3 liter (3 quart) saucepan. Add enough water just to cover.

Heat to boiling, then reduce heat to low. Cover and simmer 20 to 25 minutes or until tender. Drain, then cool slightly.

Remove sweet potato skins. Cut sweet potatoes into 1 cm (½ inch) thick slices.

Heat remaining ingredients in 10-inch frypan over medium heat, stirring constantly, until smooth and bubbly. Add sweet potatoes. Gently stir until glazed and hot.

To use these as travel snacks, roll each slice in finely chopped rolled oats (old-fashioned oats) to stop them from sticking to each other and your hands.

Cool completely before storing in an airtight plastic container in the refrigerator. To store for more than three days, freeze.

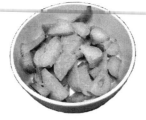

NUT FREE MUESLI BARS

> 1¼ cup rolled oats
> 1 cup puffed millet
> ½ cup unprocessed wheat bran
> ½ cup plain popcorn, unsalted [page 276]
> ½ cup toasted pearl barley [page 195]
> ¼ cup hemp seeds
> ½ teaspoon ground cardamom
> ½ teaspoon ground allspice
> 75g (5 tablespoons) unsalted HIT-friendly butter
> ¼ cup honey
> ¼ cup liquid glucose
> ½ cup brown sugar

Combine the oats, millet, bran, seeds, barley, popcorn and spices in a large bowl.

Melt the butter in a saucepan over a medium heat, then add the honey, glucose and sugar.

Bring to a boil then cook for 10 minutes, until a drop of the caramel forms a soft ball when poured into cold water.

Pour immediately over the oat mixture and beat until smooth.

Working quickly, press into a lined 27 x 18cm (10 x 7 inch) slice pan, and press flat. Set aside to cool completely before slicing with an oiled knife.

Store airtight for up to four weeks.

These muesli bars contain much less sugar and fat than most store-bought ones.

NUTTY CARAMELIZED BARLEY BITES

> **2 tablespoons brown sugar**
> **½ tablespoon light corn syrup**
> **½ tablespoon HIT-friendly butter**
> **½ cup cooked pearl barley**
> **Optional: ⅛ teaspoon ground cardamom**

Place brown sugar, corn syrup, and butter (and cardamom if you're using it) in a non-stick frypan on the stove top. Set heat to medium or medium-high. Stir the mixture as it comes together until it bubbles.

Add barley and stir to coat.

Continue cooking for 5-7 minutes, stirring constantly until barley turns golden brown in color and smells toasted.

Alternatively, after barley is coated in sugar mixture, transfer from frypan to a baking paper (parchment) lined baking tray and place in a preheated 200°C (400°F) oven.

Stir occasionally (every 1-2 minutes) until golden brown and toasted. It happens rapidly, so stay alert!

Transfer to foil, waxed paper, or parchment and cool completely. To serve, break apart with your fingers.

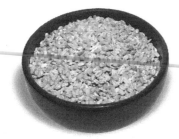

[GF] CARAMELIZED PUFFED CORN OR PUFFED RICE

> **250g (8 ounces) plain puffed corn or puffed rice**
> **1 cup HIT-friendly butter**
> **1 cup brown sugar**
> **1/2 cup light corn syrup**
> **1 teaspoon baking soda**
> **rice bran oil**
> **a pinch of salt (optional)**

Preheat oven to 120°C (250°F). Spray a large roasting dish with rice bran oil and scatter puffed corn or rice into it.

Put the butter, sugar and corn syrup into a 2 liter (2 quart) saucepan over a medium heat. Bring to bring to boil while stirring, then turn heat to low and simmer for two minutes.

Optional: If you have a sugar thermometer, cook the sugar and butter mixture to about 150 - 160°C (310 - 320°F), which is called the 'hard crack stage" for toffee and caramel. If it doesn't reach that temperature, the resulting caramel will be chewy and spongy, not crisp and hard.

Add the baking soda, and salt if using it. The caramel mixture will start to foam up. Stir well, and when mixture is blended, remove saucepan from heat.

Pour caramel mixture over puffed rice or corn in roasting dish and bake for 45 minutes, stirring every 10 -15 minutes.

Remove from oven and spread caramelized corn or rice onto baking paper to cool.

Note: You can vary the taste with a pinch of cardamom or allspice, or a teaspoon of vanilla, or by using maple syrup.

RED RHUBARB CANDY SNACKS

Storage: Any rhubarb candy, leather or fruit roll-ups should be kept in the refrigerator or freezer in an air-tight plastic bag or container. They will keep refrigerated for up to 3 weeks, and frozen for 12 months.

[GF] RHUBARB LEATHER

> **4 cups chopped red rhubarb**
> **¼ cup water**
> **2 teaspoons honey**

Place rhubarb and water in a saucepan over a medium heat. Bring mixture to a simmer until the rhubarb has begun to soften.

Let cool, and pour into a blender to make a purée.

Add 2 teaspoons of honey to the mixture. Honey and sugar helps retain the beautiful red color. You can add more if you wish, but the more sugar there is in the recipe, the longer the drying time.

Line a baking tray (cookie sheet) with plastic wrap.

Spread the purée evenly to just a ¼ inch in thickness. Make sure there is plastic showing all the way around the edge of your sheet.

The purée can be dried in a 65°C (150°F) oven, or in dehydrator.

The purée can take at least 6 - 8 hours to dry, perhaps longer.

This depends on how humid it might be, or how much sugar is in the recipe.

When the purée feels pliable, but "dryish" and not sticky, simply peel it gently from the plastic. Cut into strips, and enjoy this rhubarb-candy.

Store refrigerated, in airtight containers for up to one week, or freeze for later use.

[GF] SWEET RED RHUBARB STICKS

> **1 cup golden corn syrup**
> **2 cups water**
> **1 cup white sugar**
> **3 ½ cups of chopped red rhubarb.**

Combine the golden corn syrup, white sugar and water in a saucepan: Bring to a boil, and then add 3 ½ cups of chopped rhubarb.

Let simmer on low for 12 minutes, and remove from heat. Let the mixture stand for 30 minutes.

With a slotted spoon, remove the rhubarb pieces and place on a screen or in a colander to let the juices drip off.

Spread the rhubarb on a cookie sheet and place in a 60°C (140°F) degree oven. Let dry for at least 6 - 8 hours.

Store refrigerated, in airtight containers for 1 week or freeze for later use.

[GF] CRISP CANDIED RHUBARB STICKS

> **red rhubarb**
> **white sugar**

Simply lay thin strips of rhubarb on a parchment paper lined cookie sheet. Sprinkle them well with as much sugar as you like, and place in the oven. Set it to 80°C (180°F).

Be prepared for a drying time of at least 8 hours or more. It is also advisable to leave the oven door open to promote air circulation. Let the rhubarb dry really well, to avoid too much stickiness on the parchment paper. It could be a bit difficult to remove.

Take it out when the rhubarb is a brilliant red, crispy and kind of clear looking. Let cool completely.

[GF] CANDIED RHUBARB RIBBONS

> **1 stalk red rhubarb**
> **½ cup white sugar**
> **½ cup water**

Preheat the oven to 95°C (200°F). Line a baking tray (baking sheet) with a piece of lightly greased baking paper (parchment paper).

Using a sharp fruit and vegetable peeler or a mandoline slicer, cut the rhubarb into 15 cm (6 inch) lengths, then cut each piece into strips 0.5 to 0.3 cm (¼ to ⅛ inch) thick

Combine the sugar and water in a saucepan over high heat and bring to a boil. Cook and stir until the sugar is dissolved, then remove from the heat. Dip the rhubarb ribbons into the syrup, then place them on the prepared baking sheet, laying them out flat and ensuring that they do not touch each other.

Bake for about 45 minutes, until dry. While they are still warm, twist the strips into shapes, wrapping them around your finger or the handle of a clean wooden spoon. Use immediately, or store in an airtight container for up to 3 days.

You can use these as snacks, as a drink decoration, as topping for vanilla ice cream or as garnish for desserts such as "[GF] Mango Tart" on page 270.

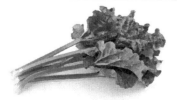

21. Beverages

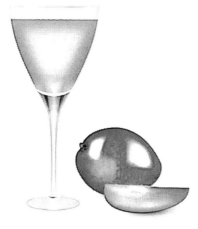

[GF] CARROT, APPLE, & BEETROOT JUICE WITH GINGER

> 7 large (about 1.2kg or 2 ½ pounds) carrots,
> peeled, topped
> 4 (about 650g or 23 ounces) beetroot bulbs,
> halved
> 4 green apples, halved
> 2 tablespoons candied ginger in syrup, drained
> crushed ice, to serve

Place all ingredients in a blender and process thoroughly. Pour into a tall glass and serve with crushed ice.

[GF] LEMONGRASS & MINT TEA

> 2 lemongrass stems, bruised, roughly chopped,
> plus extra to serve
> 2 mint sprigs, plus extra to serve
> honey, to serve

Place the lemongrass and mint in a teapot and pour over boiling water.

Leave to infuse for 10 minutes.

When ready to serve, strain the tea into glasses. Add an extra lemongrass stem as a stirrer and an extra mint sprig to each glass.

Sweeten to taste, with honey.

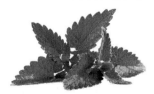

[GF] SWEET SPICED MILK

> **6-7 cardamom pods opened to the seeds**
> **6-7 whole white peppercorns,**
> **6-7 whole allspice (pimento) seeds**
> **1 cup water**
> **sugar, to taste**
> **4-6 cups HIT-friendly milk**

In a 2 liter (2 quart) saucepan, add spices to one cup of water. Bring to a boil, then remove from heat and allow to steep for 5-20 minutes, depending on how strong a spice flavor you prefer.

Add 4-6 cups of milk to the water and spices. Bring the milk and spice mixture just to a boil and remove from heat.

Add sugar. Strain into a pot. Serve, adding extra sugar or honey to taste.

[GF] HOT SPICED APPLE JUICE

> **4 apples**
> **6 whole allspice seeds and 4 cracked cardamom**
> **pods, tied in a small square of muslin**

Remove cores from apples. Cut apples into 2cm (1 inch) cubes.

Place apple and spice bag into a large saucepan. Pour five cups of cold water over them. Set saucepan over medium heat and bring to the boil.

Reduce heat to low. Simmer, partially covered with a lid, for 18 to 20 minutes or until apple is tender.

Remove spice bag and strain juice into a jug. Pour into heatproof glasses and serve.

Serves: 4

[GF] MANGO SMOOTHIE

> **400g (14 ounces) mango flesh**
> **100ml (6 ½ tablespoons) fresh apple juice**
> **270ml (9 fluid ounces) HIT-friendly milk**
> **¼ cup (70g or 2.5 ounces) whipped HIT-friendly**
> **cream**
> **1 cup ice cubes**
> **fresh mint leaves, to garnish**

Combine all ingredients in a blender and process until smooth. Pour into two tall glasses. Garnish with fresh mint leaves and serve immediately.

Serves: 2

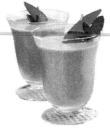

22. Sauces and Condiments

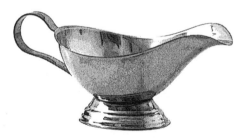

[GF] POMEGRANATE MOLASSES

> **approx. 3.5 kg (8 pounds) large, ripe pomegranates[1]**
> **¼ cup (50g or scant 2 ounces) white sugar**
>
> ---
>
> 1   If you'd rather not squeeze your own pomegranates, use 4 cups (1 liter or 1 quart) canned pomegranate juice.

It is best to juice the pomegranates by hand instead of using a juice press as the liquid from the seeds and membrane adds bitterness.

Place a large bowl into the sink (in case the juic splatters). Cut the pomegranates in half, and while squeezing the fruit with one hand, press inside the pomegranate with the fingers of the other hand, extracting as much juice as possible.

Most of the seeds will fall into the juice, so strain the juice through a sieve into another bowl and hand-squeeze the seeds in the sieve to extract every possible drop.

When you have four cups of pomegranate juice, you are ready to make molasses.

Preheat your oven to 180°C (350°F). Place a china saucer in your freezer to use for testing the consistency later on.

Pour pomegranate juice into a jug, add sugar and whisk until dissolved.

Spray rice bran oil on a a baking tray measuring 46 x 33 cm (18 x 13 inches), with a continuous lip around all four sides. This kind of tray is also called a half sheet pan.

Place the half-sheet pan in the middle rack of your preheated oven, pour the juice in and bake until it's as thick as simple syrup, about 75-80 minutes. It will thicken further as it cools, so do not let it get as thick as molasses.

To check the consistency, pour a teaspoon of it on the chilled plate and let cool in the freezer for 2 minutes. If it runs very slowly when you tilt the plate, it's done. If not, bake for another 5 minutes and repeat the test.

Pour it into a sterilized bottle (or jar), close the lid and keep in the refrigerator. It will keep in the refrigerator for at least 2 months.

Makes approximately 215g (11 tablespoons)

[GF] EXTRA RICH CARAMEL SAUCE (DAIRY FREE)

½ cup full fat HIT-friendly milk
¼ cup raw honey
2 tablespoons rice bran oil
optional: a pinch of salt

Mix all ingredients together in a small saucepan. Turn the heat to high, whisking constantly.

Once the sauce comes to a boil, lower the heat to medium.

Continue whisking constantly. When the sauce begins to thicken, turn the heat to low.

The sauce is done when the color becomes light brown. Take the saucepan off of the heat and pour the mixture into a bowl. Serve when cool.

If you need to reheat the sauce, heat on a low setting in a pot on the stove. There may be some separation of oil when reheated.

This caramel sauce is light in colour and thin and not thick.

Yield: Makes about one cup of caramel sauce.

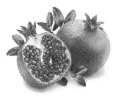

[GF] TOMATO FREE PIZZA OR PASTA SAUCE

Just keep in mind that the sauce will lose its red color the longer you cook it (beets turn brown if you over cook them) so be sure to adjust the point at which you add this tomato-less sauce to whatever you are cooking. This also means that if you freeze portions for later, be careful not to overcook when reheating.

---

1 onion, chopped
4 cloves garlic, chopped
1 cup carrots, cut into 1.5cm (½ inch) pieces
2 medium orange-fleshed sweet potatoes cubed
    (about 4 cups)
3 tablespoons fresh or frozen green mango juice[1]
½ tablespoon amchoor
salt to taste
fresh black pepper to taste
⅓ cup olive oil
230g (8 ounces) fresh baby beetroots
1 tablespoon cornflour (cornstarch)

Optional herbs:
⅓ cup chopped fresh basil or 2-3 tablespoons if
    dried
⅓ cup chopped fresh parsley or 2-3 tablespoons if
    dried
3 tablespoons chopped oregano or 2-3 teaspoons
    if dried

---

1   If this is unavailable, substitute juice of unripe apples.

In a large stock pot, sauté the onion and garlic in a little olive oil until just starting to brown.

Add the carrots, diced sweet potatoes, green mango juice, amchoor, salt and pepper then cover (barely) with water.

Bring to a boil then lower the heat and simmer (covered) for 20-30 minutes until the carrots and sweet potatoes are very soft.

Blend the contents of the pot until smooth (in batches in a blender or with an immersion blender). Add the olive oil during the blending.

The cornstarch in step 6 will thicken up the sauce slightly so don't worry if it is a little runny. If the sauce is too thick already, add some water, if too runny simmer it awhile to thicken (cover the pot but leave the lid askew).

Purée the beets and the cornstarch in a blender until very smooth, adding some water if necessary.

Add the beet mixture back to the pot and simmer for about five more minutes.

Add chopped herbs if you are using them.

Yield: approximately 6 cups of sauce.

[GF] APPLE SAUCE

2 medium granny smith apples, peeled, cored, chopped
1 tablespoon caster sugar
¼ teaspoon ground allspice
1 tablespoon ascorbic acid powder or ½ tablespoon amchoor

Place apple, sugar, allspice, ascorbic acid or amchoor and ¼ cup cold water in a saucepan over medium heat. Bring to the boil. Reduce heat to medium-low. Simmer, covered, for 10 minutes or until apple is tender.

Transfer mixture to a food processor. Process until smooth. Season with salt and pepper.

Yield: 1 ½ cups

[GF] COFFEE SYRUP

> 250 ml (8 fluid ounces) coffee
> 250g (9 ounces) sugar

Place coffee and sugar in a saucepan over a high heat. Bring the sugar and coffee mixture to a rolling boil then reduce heat to a simmer and continue to cook the mixture until it reduces and thickens into a syrup. It will have reduced enough when it thickly coats the back of a spoon.

If you reduce the syrup too much, the coffee syrup will have an unpleasant, burnt taste, so towards the end of the cooking ou will need to be particularly alert.

The syrup will last a long time if it is tightly sealed and refrigerated.

Coffee syrup can be poured over pancakes, or used to soak sponge cake or to poach fruit.

[GF] BASIC HEALTHFUL SALAD DRESSING

> **olive oil**
> **lemon-flavored herbs**
> **chopped fresh herbs, mixed**
> **salt**
> **pepper**
> **HIT-friendly cream (optional)**

Infuse your olive oil with any of the lemon-flavored herbs in our 'HIT-friendly Lemon' list.

Add a pinch of chopped, mixed herbs, some sea salt and freshly cracked black pepper.

You could also add a few scoops of HIT-friendly cream for extra ricness and smoothness.

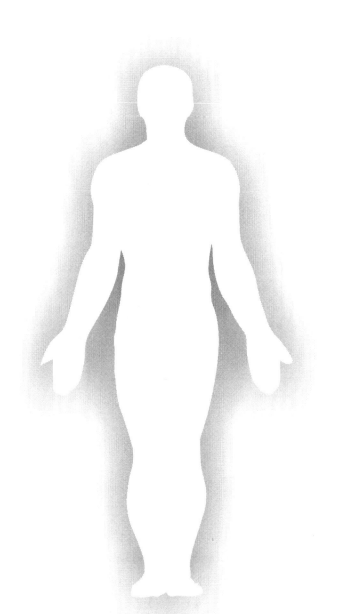

Visit the website
www.low-histamine.com

International Cookery Terms

In the U.S.A. the term 'squash' is used for the whole Cucurbita genus (family: Cucurbitaceae), including the hard-shelled winter varieties and the softer summer ones.

The term 'pumpkin' is reserved for the hard, orange-colored winter vegetable that is used to make jack-o-lanterns.

Other varieties of squash are referred to specifically—as acorn squash, zucchini, patty pan, kuri, butternut and so on.

Below is a brief guide to some more international cookery terms.

AUSTRALIA	U.K.	U.S.A.
baking paper	baking paper	parchment paper
baking tray	baking tray	baking sheet
beetroot	beetroot	beet
bicarbonate of soda or bicarb soda	bicarbonate of soda or bicarb soda	baking soda
biscuit	biscuit	cookie
bread flour	strong flour	bread flour
butternut pumpkin	butternut pumpkin	butternut squash
cake tin	cake tin	cake baking pan
cantaloupe	rockmelon	cantaloupe
capsicum	capsicum	sweet or bell pepper

AUSTRALIA	U.K.	U.S.A.
castor sugar or caster sugar	castor sugar	superfine sugar or caster sugar
celery stick	celery stick	celery rib
chips or potato chips	crisps	chips or potato chips
chips	chips	fries or French fries
coriander	coriander	cilantro
cornflour	cornflour	corn starch
cornmeal	maize flour	cornmeal
dessert	pudding	dessert
eggplant	aubergine	eggplant
frying pan	frying pan	skillet, frying pan or frypan
glacé fruits	glacé fruits	candied fruit
greaseproof paper	greaseproof paper	wax paper
green beans	French beans	green beans
ground coriander	coriander seed	coriander
hard-boiled egg	hard-boiled egg	hard-cooked egg
icing sugar	icing sugar	confectioners' sugar or powdered sugar
jam	jam	jelly
Japanese pumpkin		kabocha squash
jelly	jelly	jell-o
loaf tin	loaf tin	loaf pan
minced meat	minced meat	ground meat
pastry	pastry	pie crust
plain flour	plain flour	all purpose flour
reduced fat cream	single cream	light cream or half-and-half

AUSTRALIA	U.K.	U.S.A.
rice flour	ground rice	rice flour
rich cream or double cream	double cream	heavy cream
roquette or rocket	roquette or rocket	arugula
scone	scone	biscuit
self-raising flour	self-raising flour	self-rising flour
semolina	semolina	farina
sieve or strainer	sieve	strainer
silver beet	silver beet	Swiss chard
spring onion	spring onion or salad onion	scallion or green onion
summer squash		patty-pan squash
swede	swede or swede turnip (known in Scotland as 'turnip' or 'neep')	rutabaga
tea towel	tea towel	dish towel
to sift	to sift	to strain
tomato sauce	tomato sauce	catsup, ketchup
vanilla bean or vanilla pod	vanilla pod	vanilla bean
zucchini	zucchini	courgette

GLOSSARY

DOUBLE BLIND

This is an experimental procedure in which neither the subjects of the experiment nor the persons administering the experiment know the critical aspects of the experiment; "a double-blind procedure is used to guard against both experimenter bias and placebo effects". [200]

FOOD CHALLENGE

This is a process of testing for food allergies in which the patient is given, often in double-blind conditions, a sample of a different, potentially allergenic, food once a day and reactions are noted. In some forms the challenge is preceded by a diet from which all common allergens have been eliminated for several weeks, after which foods are introduced as above. [199]

H1 RECEPTOR ANTAGONISTS

H1 antihistamines are clinically used in the treatment of histamine-mediated allergic conditions. To be specific, these indications may include:

Allergic rhinitis
Allergic conjunctivitis
Allergic dermatological conditions (contact dermatitis)

Rhinorrhea (runny nose)
Urticaria
Angioedema
Diarrhea
Pruritus (atopic dermatitis, insect bites)
Anaphylactic or anaphylactoid reactions—adjunct only
Nausea and vomiting
Sedation (first-generation H1-antihistamines)

H1-antihistamines can be administered topically (through the skin, nose, or eyes) or systemically, based on the nature of the allergic condition. [195]

H2 RECEPTOR ANTAGONISTS

The H2 receptor antagonists are a class of drugs used to block the action of histamine on parietal cells (specifically the histamine H2 receptors) in the stomach, decreasing the production of acid by these cells. H2 antagonists are used in the treatment of dyspepsia, although they have been surpassed in popularity by the more effective proton pump inhibitors.

The prototypical H2 antagonist was cimetidine, ... first marketed in 1976.

H2-antagonists are used by clinicians in the treatment of acid-related gastrointestinal conditions, including:
Peptic ulcer disease (PUD)
Gastroesophageal reflux disease (GERD/GORD)
Dyspepsia
Prevention of stress ulcer (a specific indication of ranitidine)

People who suffer from infrequent heartburn may take either antacids or H2-receptor antagonists for treatment. The H2-antagonists offer several advantages over antacids. ... Proton pump inhibitors, however, are the preferred treatment for erosive esophagitis since they have been shown to promote healing better than H2-antagonists.

Histamine H2 receptor blockers may have therapeutic benefits for CHF by blocking the action of histamine in the heart.

The H2 antagonist Ranitidine is prescribed by some urologists for patients with interstitial cystitis. Interstitial cystitis (IC) patients have been found to have significantly more mast cells than non-IC individuals. Mast cells explode with histamine. Studies have suggested that antihistamines improve IC-related pelvic pain. [196]

H3 RECEPTOR ANTAGONISTS

An H3-receptor antagonist is a classification of drugs used to block the action of histamine at the H3 receptor.

Unlike the H1 and H2 receptors which have primarily peripheral actions, but cause sedation if they are blocked in the brain, H3 receptors are primarily found in the brain and are inhibitory autoreceptors located on histaminergic nerve terminals, which modulate the release of histamine.

Histamine release in the brain triggers secondary release of excitatory neurotransmitters such as glutamate and acetylcholine via stimulation of H1 receptors in the cerebral cortex. Consequently unlike the H1 antagonist antihistamines which are sedating, H3 antagonists have stimulant and nootropic effects, and are being researched as potential drugs for the treatment of neurodegenerative conditions such as Alzheimer's disease. [197]

H4 RECEPTOR ANTAGONISTS

By inhibiting the H4 receptor, asthma and allergy may be treated. The highly selective histamine H4 antagonist VUF-6002 is orally active and inhibits the activity of both mast cells and eosinophils in vivo, and has antiinflammatory and antihyperalgesic effects. [198]

HISTADELIA

'Histadelia is an inherited condition characterized by elevated blood levels of histamine. Histamine excess can be manifest as asthma, vasomotor rhinitis, allergic skin disorders with pruritis, excess stomach acid production, saliva, tears, and thin nasal and bronchial secretions, and certain types of vascular headaches.

'For some individuals, high levels of blood histamine have psychological, behavioral, and cognitive symptoms. 15-20% of schizophrenics and many suffers of depression may have histadelia. Suffers may be suicidally depressed and fall prey to obsessions, compulsions, and addictions.

'Other symptoms include: good tolerance of cold, poor tolerance of heat, unexplained nausea, poor pain tolerance, excess/abundant saliva in mouth, frequent colds/flu, phobias, highly motivated and hard-driving personality, good creativity/ imagination, high libido, joint pain/swelling/stiffness, excess perspiration, warm skin. Histamine speeds up metabolism producing a tendency towards hyperactivity.' [201]

SAGO

"Sago' is a starch extracted from the pith, or middle part, of the trunk of a tropical Sago Palm (Metroxylon sagu) or similar species of palm such as Metroxylon warburgii. The trunk of some cycads such as Cycas circinalis are also used for what is called 'sago'. [187]

Sago is almost pure carbohydrate. It is low in fat but high in calories, and not a good source of protein and fiber. Neither does it contain many vitamins and minerals.

Sago starch can be baked (resulting in a product comparable to bread, biscuits or pancakes) or combined with boiling water to make a paste. Food manufacturers use it to make noodles and white bread. Powdered sago may be added as a thickener for other dishes, or used as a dense flour. Sago flour is often a main ingredient in steamed puddings such as sago plum pudding.

Pearl sago closely resembles *pearl tapioca.* 'Both are usually small (approximately 2 mm. in diameter) dry, opaque balls, typically white. When they are soaked and cooked, both pearl sago pearl tapioca swell, becoming bigger, softer and translucent. Both are popular in Indian, Bangladeshi and Sri Lankan cuisine and all over the world. In western cookery they are usually used to make puddings.

Bibliography

[1] Marieb, E. (2001). Human anatomy & physiology. San Francisco: Benjamin Cummings. p. 414.

[2] Noszal, B.; Kraszni, M.; Racz, A. (2004). "Histamine: fundamentals of biological chemistry". In Falus, A.; Grosman, N.; Darvas, Z. Histamine: Biology and Medical Aspects. Budapest: Spring-Med. pp. 15–28.

[3] Di Giuseppe, M., et al. (2003). Nelson Biology 12. Toronto: Thomson Canada. p. 473.

[4] Hancock AA. H3 receptor antagonists/inverse agonists as anti-obesity agents. Curr Opin Investig Drugs. 2003 Oct;4(10):1190-7.

[5] Gupta, Meera et al., Research Article 658. Antiallergic impact of aloe vera extract on dye wastewater treated Swiss albino rats. Indian Journal of Fundamental and Applied Life Sciences ISSN: 2231 - 6345 2013 Vol. 3 (3) July - September, pp. 658 - 661

[6] Komericki P, et al. Histamine intolerance: lack of reproducibility of single symptoms by oral provocation with histamine: a randomised, double-blind, placebo-controlled cross-over study. Wiener klinische Wochenschrift, January 2011, Volume 123, Issue 1-2, pp 15-20

[7]Sattler J, Häfner D, Klotter HJ, Lorenz W, Wagner PK. Food-induced histaminosis as an epidemiological problem: plasma histamine elevation and haemodynamic alterations after oral histamine administration and blockade of diamine oxidase (DAO). Agents and Actions. 1988 Apr;23(3-4):361-5.

[8]Ede, Georgia, MD. Diagnosis: Diet. Freshness Counts: Histamine Intolerance. 2013. Retrieved January 2014.

[9]Teta, Dr Jillian Sarno. A Different Type of Food Sensitivity, Histamine Intolerance. fixyourdigestion.com accessed January 2014.

[10]   Baker, Dr Jillian. A study of antagonist affinities for the human histamine H2 receptor. Br J Pharmacol. 2008 Mar;153(5):1011-21. Epub 2007 Dec 24.

[11]   Maintz, Laura & Novak, Natalija. Histamine and histamine intolerance. American Journal of Clinical Nutrition. May 2007 vol. 85 no. 5 1185-1196

[12]   Lawley, Richard. Scombrotoxin (Histamine). foodsafetywatch.org, January 30, 2013. Retrieved January 2014.

[13]   Moyer, Melinda Wenner. Nothing to Sneeze At: Allergies May Be Good for You, Scientific American, June 1, 2012.

[14]   Brook, R.D. et al., Particulate Matter Air Pollution and Cardiovascular Disease, An Update to the Scientific Statement From the American Heart Association. Circulation. 2010 Jun 1;121(21):2331-78. doi: 10.1161/CIR.0b013e3181dbece1. Epub 2010 May 10.

[15]   Martin Metz et al., Evidence for Non-Allergic Mast Cell Activation in Pollen-Associated Inflammation. Journal of Investigative Dermatology (2011) 131, 987–990; doi:10.1038/jid.2010.419; published online 20 January 2011.

[16]   Seo, Makoto et al. Immunotoxic Effects of Trichloroethylene and Tetrachloroethylene. Journal of Health Science, 57(6)
488–496 (2011)

[17]   Joneja, Dr. J. V., Dietary Management of Food Allergies &
Intolerances: A Comprehensive Guide. J. A. Hall Publications,
1998.

[18]   Taylor, S.L., Stratton, J.E. & Hutkins, R.W. Biogenic amines
in cheese and other fermented foods: a review. J. Food Prot.
54:460-470, 1991.

[19]   Naila, Aishath et al. Control of Biogenic Amines in Food—
Existing and Emerging Approaches. J Food Sci. 2010 September;
75(7): R139–R150.

[20]   Lewis, Robert Alan (1998). Lewis' Dictionary of Toxicol-
ogy. CRC Press. p. 212. ISBN 1-56670-223-2.

[21]   Nowotarski, S.L. et al—2013   Polyamines and cancer:
implications for chemotherapy and chemoprevention. Expert
Reviews in Molecular Medicine (Impact Factor: 6.62). 01/2013;
15:e3. DOI:10.1017/erm.2013.3

[22]   Scully, Professor Crispian. 'Diet Free of Cinnamon and
Benzoates.' The British Society for Oral Medicine. Patient Information: Patient Information Leaflets. February 2005

[23]   Cimbollek, S. et al, NSAID-Sensitive Antihistamine-
Induced Urticaria/Angioedema. J Investig Allergol Clin
Immunol. 2011;21(6):488-90.

[24]   Baldo BA, Pham NH. Histamine-releasing and allergenic
properties of opioid analgesic drugs: resolving the two. Anaesth
Intensive Care. 2012 Mar;40(2):216-35.

[25]   Van Auken, Candace. Histamine — Beyond mast cells.
Idiopathic anaphylaxis information center. www.iainfoctr.com
Retrieved January 2014

[26]   Baldwin AL. Mast cell activation by stress. Methods Mol Biol. 2006;315:349-60.

[27]   Eutamene H. Acute stress modulates the histamine content of mast cells in the gastrointestinal tract through interleukin-1 and corticotropin-release in rats. J Physiol. 553(Pt 3). 959-966. 2003.

[28]   Shah, Shilpa. Hormonal Link to Autoimmune Allergies. ISRN Allergy Volume 2012 (2012), Article ID 910437.

[29]   A. Haeggström, A. B. Östberg, P. Stjerna, P. Graf, and H. Hallén. Nasal mucosal swelling and reactivity during a menstrual cycle. ORL Journal for Oto-Rhino-Laryngology and Its Related Specialties, vol. 62, no. 1, pp. 39–42, 2000.

[30]   Hyman, Mark, MD. Maximizing Methylation: The Key to Healthy Aging. http://drhyman.com February 8, 2011. Retrived January 2014.

[31]   Maintz L, Benfadal S, Allam JP, Hagemann T, Fimmers R, Novak N. Evidence for a reduced histamine degradation capacity in a subgroup of patients with atopic eczema. J Allergy Clin Immunol. 2006 May;117(5):1106-12. Epub 2006 Feb 8.

[32]   Guita, Mahendm Kumar, M.D., et al. Histamine - can It Cause An Acute Coronary Event? Clinical Cardiology 24, 258-259 (2001)

[33]   Dechene L. Chronic fatigue syndrome: influence of histamine, hormones and electrolytes. Med Hypotheses. 40(1). 55-60. 1993. Jan;40(1):55-60.

[34]   Blanco I, Béritze N, Argüelles M, Cárcaba V, Fernández F, Janciauskiene S, Oikonomopoulou K, de Serres FJ, Fernández-Bustillo E, Hollenberg MD. Abnormal overexpression of mastocytes in skin biopsies of fibromyalgia patients. Clin Rheumatol. 2010 Dec;29(12):1403-12. doi: 10.1007/s10067-010-1474-7. Epub 2010 Apr 30.

[35]   M Taweevisit, N Wisadeopas, U Phumsuk, P S Thorner. Increased mast cell density in haemorrhoid venous blood vessels suggests a role in pathogenesis. Singapore medical journal (Impact Factor: 0.63). 0½2009; 49(12):977-9. Source: PubMed.

[36]   Hasturk H, Kantarci A, Ebrahimi N, Andry C, Holick M, Jones VL, Van Dyke TE. Topical H2 antagonist prevents periodontitis in a rabbit model. Infect Immun. 2006 Apr;74(4):2402-14.

[37]   Lukasik E., et al. Cryotherapy decreases histamine levels in the blood of patients with rheumatoid arthritis. Inflamm Res. 2010 Mar;59 Suppl 2:S253-5. doi: 10.1007/s00011-009-0144-1.

[38]   Fox CC, Lichtenstein LM, Roche JK. Intestinal mast cell responses in idiopathic inflammatory bowel disease. Histamine release from human intestinal mast cells in response to gut epithelial proteins. Dig Dis Sci. 1993 Jun;38(6):1105-12.

[39]   Torrealba F, et al. Histamine and motivation. Front Syst Neurosci. 2012 Jul 4;6:51. doi: 10.3389/fnsys.2012.00051.

[40]   Jadidi-Niaragh F, Mirshafiey A. Histamine and histamine receptors in pathogenesis and treatment of multiple sclerosis. Neuropharmacology. 2010 Sep;59(3):180-9. doi: 10.1016/j.neuropharm.2010.05.005. Epub 2010 May 21.

[41]   Ramras, Donald G. MD., Scombroid Poisoning from Mahi-Mahi. West J Med. 1974 November; 121(5): 415–416.

[42]   Smart DR. Scombroid poisoning. A report of seven cases involving the Western Australian salmon, Arripis truttaceus. Med J Aust. 1992 Dec 7-21;157(11-12):748-51.

[43]   Lawley, Richard. Scombrotoxin (histamine). Food Safety Watch, January 30, 2013

[44]   Taylor SL, Stratton JE, Nordlee JA. Histamine poisoning (scombroid fish poisoning): an allergy-like intoxication. J Toxicol Clin Toxicol. 1989;27(4-5):225-40.

[45]   Lewiecki, E. Michael M.D., Osteoporosis: Clinical Evaluation. Endotext Clinical Endocrinology. Updated: November 28,
2010.

[46]   Kinjo M, Setoguchi S, Solomon DH. Antihistamine therapy
and bone mineral density: analysis in a population-based US
sample. Am J Med. 2008 Dec;121(12):1085-91. doi: 10.1016/j.
amjmed.2008.06.036.

[47]   Prado RF, Silveira VÁ, Rocha RF, Vasconcellos LM, Carv-
alho YR. Effects of experimental osteoporosis and low calcium
intake on postextraction sockets of rats. Int J Exp Pathol. 2012
Apr;93(2):139-47. doi: 10.1111/j.1365-2613.2012.00809.x. Epub
2012 Feb 24.

[48]   Chiappetta, Nicole DO, and Gruber, Barry MD. The Role of
Mast Cells in Osteoporosis. Seminars in Arthritis and Rheuma-
tism 2006 Aug;36(1):32-6. Epub 2006 Jul 3.

[49]   Naddafi, Fatemeh MSc & Mirshafiey, Abbas PhD. The
Neglected Role of Histamine in Alzheimer's Disease. Am J
Alzheimers Dis Other Demen May 15, 2013 1533317513488925

[50]   Nuutinen S, Panula P. Histamine in neurotransmission and
brain diseases. Adv Exp Med Biol. 2010;709:95-107.

[51]   Das, Undurti N. Molecular Basis of Health and Disease.
ISBN: 9789400704954 Publication Date: 2013-09-29 Publisher:
Springer Netherlands.

[52]   Lin, Jian-Sheng et al., Histamine H3 Receptors and Sleep-
Wake Regulation. Published online before print September 23,
2010, doi: 10.1124/jpet.110.170134 JPET January 2011 vol. 336
no. 1 17-23

[53]   Kuo, CH; Pang, L; Chang, R. Vertigo-part 2-management
in general practice. Australian family physician 37 (6): 409–413.
PMID 18523693. (June 2008)

[54]   Wikipedia: Motion Sickness, retrieved January 2014.

[55]   Kimura K, Rüsch D, Strasser C, Lengkong M, Wulf H, Koller M, Celik I. Influence of histamine release on postoperative vomiting (POV) following gynaecological laparoscopic surgery. Inflamm Res. 2004 Aug;53 Suppl 2:S148-53. Epub 2004 Aug 10.

[56]   Shaw, Graham G. Hypothermia produced in mice by histamine acting on the central nervous system. Br J Pharmacol. 1971 June; 42(2): 205–214.

[57]   Bugajski J, Zacny E. The role of central histamine H1- and H2-receptors in hypothermia induced by histamine in the rat. Agents Actions. 1981 Nov;11(5):442-7.

[58]   Onodera K, Shinoda H, Watanabe T. Effects of thiamine administration on hypothermia and hypothalamic histamine levels in dietary-induced thiamine deficient rats. Jpn J Pharmacol. 1990 Nov;54(3):339-43.

[59]   von Rahden BH, Jurowich C, Kircher S, Lazariotou M, Jung M, Germer CT, Grimm M. Allergic predisposition, histamine and histamine receptor expression (H1R, H2R) are associated with complicated courses of sigmoid diverticulitis. J Gastrointest Surg. 2012 Jan;16(1):173-82; discussion 182. doi: 10.1007/s11605-011-1702-8. Epub 2011 Sep 29.

[60]   Meniere's Australia, Resource and Information Centre, retrived January 2014

[61]   Lacour, Michel et al., Betahistine in the treatment of Ménière's disease. Neuropsychiatr Dis Treat. 2007 August; 3(4): 429–440.

[62]   Henderson, Karin & David. Histamine and Antihistamines: What It Is, How It Works And How It Relates To Ménière's Disease Symptoms. Ménière's-disease.ca Information and Resources. British Columbia, Canada. Retrieved January 2014.

[63]   Esposito, Pamela et al., Acute stress increases permeability of the blood–brain-barrier through activation of brain mast cells. Brain Research 888 (2001) 117–127

[64]   Sarker MH, Easton AS, Fraser PA. Regulation of cerebral microvascular permeability by histamine in the anaesthetized rat. J Physiol. 1998 Mar 15;507 (Pt 3):909-18.

[65]   H Nolte, H. et al., Histamine release from gut mast cells from patients with inflammatory bowel diseases. Gut. 1990 July; 31(7): 791–794.

[66]   Wake, Hidenori et al., Histamine Inhibits Advanced Glycation End Products-Induced Adhesion Molecule Expression on Human Monocytes. Journal of Pharmacology and Experimental Therapeutics 2009 Sep;330(3):826-33. doi: 10.1124/jpet.109.155960. Epub 2009 Jun 30.

[67]   Yanai, K; Tashiro, M (2007). "The physiological and pathophysiological roles of neuronal histamine: an insight from human positron emission tomography studies.". Pharmacology & therapeutics 113 (1): 1–15. doi:10.1016/j.pharmthera.2006.06.008. PMID 16890992.

[68]   Alvarez, EO (2009). "The role of histamine on cognition.". Behavioural Brain Research 199 (2): 183–9. doi:10.1016/j.bbr.2008.12.010. PMID 19126417.

[69]   Ito, C (2004). "The role of the central histaminergic system on schizophrenia". Drug News & Perspectives 17 (6): 383–7. doi:10.1358/dnp.2004.17.6.829029. PMID 15334189.

[70]   Alvarez, EO (2009). "The role of histamine on cognition.". Behavioural Brain Research 199 (2): 183–9. doi:10.1016/j.bbr.2008.12.010. PMID 19126417.

[71]   van Ruitenbeek, P, & Mehta, M A. Potential enhancing effects of histamine H1 agonism/H3 antagonism on working memory assessed by performance and bold response in healthy volunteers. Br J Pharmacol. 2013 Sep;170(1):144-55. doi: 10.1111/bph.12184.

[72]   White, JM; Rumbold, GR (1988). "Behavioural effects of histamine and its antagonists: a review.". Psychopharmacology 95 (1): 1-14. PMID 3133686.

[73]   Cará, AM; Lopes-Martins, RA; Antunes, E; Nahoum, CR; De Nucci, G (1995). "The role of histamine in human penile erection.". British Journal of Urology 75 (2): 220-4. doi:10.1111/ j.1464-410X.1995.tb07315.x. PMID 7850330.

[74]   White, JM; Rumbold, GR (1988). "Behavioural effects of histamine and its antagonists: a review.". Psychopharmacology 95 (1): 1-14. PMID 3133686.

[75]   DeVault KR, Castell DO (1999). "Updated guidelines for the diagnosis and treatment of gastroesophageal reflux disease. The Practice Parameters Committee of the American College of Gastroenterology". Am J Gastroenterol 94 (6): 1434-42. doi:10.1111/j.1572-0241.1999.1123_a.x. PMID 10364004.

[76]   What Types of Drugs Treat GERD? WebMD. Sourced from National Digestive Diseases Information Clearing House: Heartburn, Gastroesophageal Reflux (GER), and Gastroesophageal Reflux Disease (GERD)

[77]   Mandler, George. Why Acid Reflux Medication May Be Harmful. http://iwellnesscenter.com Wednesday, March 2nd, 2011. Retrieved January 2014

[78]   Russell RM, Golner BB, Krasinski SD, Sadowski JA, Suter PM, Braun CL. Effect of antacid and H2 receptor antagonists on the intestinal absorption of folic acid. J Lab Clin Med. 1988 Oct;112(4):458-63.

[79]   Theoharides TC, Sismanopoulos N, Delivanis DA, Zhang B, Hatziagelaki EE, Kalogeromitros D. Mast cells squeeze the heart and stretch the gird: Their role in atherosclerosis and obesity. Trends Pharmacol Sci. 2011 Sep;32(9):534-42. doi: 10.1016/j.tips.2011.05.005. Epub 2011 Jul 7.

[80]   Kennedy, Lindsey et al., Histamine and histamine receptor regulation of gastrointestinal cancers. Translational Gastrointestinal Cancer, Vol 1, No 3 (October 2012)

[81]   Falus A, Pós Z, Darvas Z. Histamine in normal and malignant cell proliferation. Adv Exp Med Biol. 2011;709:109-23. doi: 10.^{1007}/$_{978}$-1-4419-8056-4_11.

[82]   Medina, Vanina A. et al., Histamine Receptors as Potential Therapeutic Targets for Cancer Drug Development. ^{12}/$_{2011}$; ISBN: 978-953-307-257-9 In book: Drug Development—A Case Study Based Insight into Modern Strategies.

[83]   Joneja, Dr Janice. Histamine intolerance. Action Against Allergy newsletter, March 2010

[84]   Bodmer S, Imark C, Kneubühl M. Biogenic amines in foods: histamine and food processing. Inflamm Res. 1999 Jun;48(6):296-300.

[85]   Ede, Georgia MD. Freshness Counts: Histamine Intolerance. March 2013 www.diagnosisdiet.com/histamine-intolerance/ Retrieved January 2014

[86]   Tinajero, Lori Ann. Food Allergies may be simply a DAO deficiency. East Valley Holistic Health Examiner. October 19, 2010

[87]   Malone, Marilyn H.; Metcalfe, Dean D. Histamine in Foods: Its Possible Role in Non-Allergic Adverse Reactions to Ingestants. Allergy and Asthma Proceedings, Volume 7, Number 3, May-June 1986 , pp. 241-245(5)

[88]   Johnston CS. The antihistamine action of ascorbic acid. Subcellular Biochemistry 1996;25:189–213.

[89]   Ji Y, Sakata Y, Tso P. Nutrient-induced inflammation in the intestine. Curr Opin Clin Nutr Metab Care. 2011 Jul;14(4):315-21. doi: 10.1097/MCO.0b013e3283476e74.

[90]   Ji Y, Sakata Y, Li X, Zhang C, Yang Q, Xu M, Wollin A, Langhans W, Tso P. Lymphatic diamine oxidase secretion stimulated by fat absorption is linked with histamine release. American Journal of Physiology—Gastrointestinal and Liver Physiology. 2013 Apr 15;304(8):G732-40. doi: 10.1152/ajpgi.00399.2012. Epub 2013 Feb 14.

[91]   Schaubschläger WW, Becker WM, Schade U, Zabel P, Schlaak M. Release of mediators from human gastric mucosa and blood in adverse reactions to benzoate. Int Arch Allergy Appl Immunol. 1991;96(2):97-101.

[92]   Mio M, Yabuta M, Kamei C. Ultraviolet B (UVB) light-induced histamine release from rat peritoneal mast cells and its augmentation by certain phenothiazine compounds. Immunopharmacology. 1999 Jan;41(1):55-63.

[93]   Malaviya, Rama et al., Histamine in Human Epidermal Cells is Induced by Ultraviolet Light Injury. Journal of Investigative Dermatology (1996) 106, 785–789; doi:10.1111/1523-1747. ep12346356

[94]   Wojciech Barg, Wojciech Medrala, and Anna Wolanczyk-Medrala. Exercise-Induced Anaphylaxis: An Update on Diagnosis and Treatment. Curr Allergy Asthma Rep. 2011 February; 11(1): 45–51. Published online 2010 October 5. doi: 10.1007/s11882-010-0150-y

[95]   Gelfand, Jodi. Alternatives to antihistamines. www.drhoffman.com, retrieved January 2014.

[96]　Pavan, Rajendra; Jain, Sapna; Shraddha and Kumar, Ajay. Properties and Therapeutic Application of Bromelain: A Review. Biotechnology Research International. Volume 2012 (2012), Article ID 976203, 6 pages. http://dx.doi.org/10.1155/2012/976203

[97]　Johnston CS, Martin LJ, Cai X. Antihistamine effect of supplemental ascorbic acid and neutrophil chemotaxis. J Am Coll Nutr. 1992 Apr;11(2):172-6.

[98]　Johnston CS, Solomon RE, Corte C (December 1996). "Vitamin C depletion is associated with alterations in blood histamine and plasma free carnitine in adults". J Am Coll Nutr 15 (6): 586–91. PMID 8951736.

[99]　Clemetson CA (April 1980). "Histamine and ascorbic acid in human blood". J. Nutr. 110 (4): 662–8. PMID 7365537.

[100]　Johnston C. et al. Antihistamine effect of supplemental ascorbic acid and neutrophil chemotaxis" J Am Coll Nutr 11 (1992):172-76.

[101]　Force RW, Nahata MC. Effect of histamine H2-receptor antagonists on vitamin B12 absorption. Ann Pharmacother. 1992 Oct;26(10):1283-6.

[102]　Ruscin JM, Page RL 2nd, Valuck RJ. Vitamin B(12) deficiency associated with histamine(2)-receptor antagonists and a proton-pump inhibitor. Ann Pharmacother. 2002 May;36(5):812-6.

[103]　Russell RM, Golner BB, Krasinski SD, Sadowski JA, Suter PM, Braun CL. Effect of antacid and H2 receptor antagonists on the intestinal absorption of folic acid. J Lab Clin Med. 1988 Oct;112(4):458-63.

[104]　Goodhart, Robert S. & Shils, Maurice E. (1980). Modern Nutrition in Health and Disease (6th ed.). Philadelphia: Lea and Febinger. pp. 134–138. ISBN 0-8121-0645-8.

[105]   Fattahi, Mohammad Javad & Mirshafiey, Abbas. Pros-
taglandins and Rheumatoid Arthritis. Hindawi. Arthritis.
Volume 2012 (2012), Article ID 239310, 7 pages. http://dx.doi.
org/10.^{1155}/$_{2012}$/239310

[106]   Ehrlich, Steven D. NMD. Omega-3 fatty acids. University of
Maryland Medical Center health information, ^{05}/$_{10}$/2011.

[107]   Kris-Etherton, Penny. Lyon Diet Heart Study. Benefits of a
Mediterranean-Style, National Cholesterol Education Program/
American Heart Association Step I Dietary Pattern on Cardio-
vascular Disease. Circulation. 2001; 103: 1823-1825 doi: 10.^{1161}/
^{01}.CIR.103.13.1823

[108]   Author unknown. Melrose Organic Flaxseed Oil. Melrose
Laboratories Pty Ltd. www.melrosehealth.com.au, retrieved January 2014

[109]   Whitney, Ellie and Rolfes, SR (2008). Understanding Nutrition (11th ed.). California: Thomson Wadsworth. p. 154.

[110]   Burr, G.O., Burr, M.M. and Miller, E. (1930). On the nature
and role of the fatty acids essential in nutrition. (PDF). J. Biol.
Chem. 86 (587). Retrieved 2007-01-17.

[111]   Author unknown. A Danish Expert Finds Flaxseed and
Other Plant Oils Simply Better than Fish and Krill. Fatty Acids
Hub. Retrieved 2011-04-01.

[112]   Legleiter, L. R. and Spears, J. W. Plasma diamine oxidase: A
biomarker of copper deficiency in the bovine. J Anim Sci. 2007
Sep;85(9):2198-204. Epub 2007 May 25.

[113]   Jones AA, DiSilvestro RA, Coleman M, Wagner TL. Copper
supplementation of adult men: effects on blood copper enzyme
activities and indicators of cardiovascular disease risk. Metabolism. 1997 Dec;46(12):1380-3.

[114] Lands, WEM (2005). Fish, Omega 3 and human health. American Oil Chemists' Society. ISBN 978-1-893997-81-3.

[115] Polovic N, Blanusa M, Gavrovic-Jankulovic M, Atanas-kovic-Markovic M, Burazer L, Jankov R, Cirkovic Velickovic T.

[116] A matrix effect in pectin-rich fruits hampers digestion of allergen by pepsin in vivo and in vitro. Clin Exp Allergy. 2007 May;37(5):764-71.

[117] Choi SP, Kang MY, Koh HJ, Nam SH, Friedman M. Antiallergic activities of pigmented rice bran extracts in cell assays. J Food Sci. 2007 Nov;72(9):S719-26.

[118] Justia Patents, Patent Application (Application #20130171280)

[119] Sun Phil Choi, Sung Phil Kim, Mi Young Kang, Seok Hyun Nam, and Mendel Friedman. Protective Effects of Black Rice Bran against Chemically-Induced Inflammation of Mouse Skin. Journal of Agricultural and Food Chemistry 2010 58 (18), 10007-10015

[120] ACS News Service Weekly PressPac: Black Rice Bran May Help Fight Disease-Related Inflammation." American Chemical Society. ACS, 20 Oct. 2010. Web. 11 Nov. 2010.

[121] Marone G, Columbo M, de Paulis A, Cirillo R, Giugliano R, Condorelli M. Physiological concentrations of zinc inhibit the release of histamine from human basophils and lung mast cells. Agents Actions. 1986 Apr;18(1-2):103-6.

[122] Chakravarty N. & Yu WJ. Regulatory role of calcium on histamine secretion. Agents Actions. 1986 Apr;18(1-2):57-60.

[123] Bois, P., Gascon, A. & Beaulnes, A. Histamine-liberating Effect of Magnesium Deficiency in the Rat. Nature 197, 501 - 502 (02 February 1963); doi:10.^{1038}/197501a0.

[124]   Nishio A, Ishiguro S, Miyao N. Specific change of histamine metabolism in acute magnesium-deficient young rats. Drug Nutr Interact. 1987;5(2):89-96.

[125]   Thomas, Carissa M. et al. Histamine Derived from Probiotic Lactobacillus reuteri Suppresses TNF via Modulation of PKA and ERK Signaling. PLOS One. Published: February 22, 2012. DOI: 10.1371/journal.pone.0031951

[126]   E. Schiavi, et al. Oral therapeutic administration of a probiotic mixture suppresses established Th2 responses and systemic anaphylaxis in a murine model of food allergy. Article first published online: 8 NOV 2010. DOI: 10.1111/j.1398-9995.2010.02501.x © 2010 John Wiley & Sons A/S

[127]   Oksaharju A, Kankainen M, Kekkonen RA, Lindstedt KA, Kovanen PT, Korpela R, Miettinen M. Probiotic Lactobacillus rhamnosus downregulates FCER1 and HRH4 expression in human mast cells. World J Gastroenterol. 2011 Feb 14;17(6):750-9. doi: 10.3748/wjg.v17.i6.750.

[128]   Hyo-Hyun Park, et al. Flavonoids inhibit histamine release and expression of proinflammatory cytokines in mast cells. Pharmacal Research. October 2008, Volume 31, Issue 10, pp 1303-1311

[129]   Theoharides TC, Kempuraj D, Iliopoulou BP. Mast cells, T cells, and inhibition by luteolin: implications for the pathogenesis and treatment of multiple sclerosis. Adv Exp Med Biol. 2007;601:423-30.

[130]   Wikipedia: Luteolin. Retrieved January 2014

[131]   Asthma. University of Maryland Medical Center. Retrieved 2013-06-21

[132]   Deng GF, Xu XR, Zhang Y, Li D, Gan RY, Li HB. Phenolic compounds and bioactivities of pigmented rice. Crit Rev Food Sci Nutr. 2013;53(3):296-306. doi: 10.^{1080}/$_{10408398}$.2010.529624.

[133]   Stewart LK, Soileau JL, Ribnicky D, Wang ZQ, Raskin I, Poulev A, Majewski M, Cefalu WT, Gettys TW (July 2008). "Quercetin transiently increases energy expenditure but persistently decreases circulating markers of inflammation in C57BL/6J mice fed a high-fat diet". Metab. Clin. Exp. 57 (7 Suppl 1): S39–46. doi:10.1016/j.metabol.2008.03.003. PMC 2596873. PMID 18555853.

[134]   Jung, Min Kyung; Hur, Dae Young; Song, Seok Bean; Park, Yoorim; Kim, Tae Sung; Bang, Sa Ik; Kim, Seonghan; Song, Hyun Keun; Park, Hyunjeong; Cho, Dae Ho (2010). "Tannic Acid and Quercetin Display a Therapeutic Effect in Atopic Dermatitis via Suppression of Angiogenesis and TARC Expression in Nc/Nga Mice". Journal of Investigative Dermatology 130 (5): 1459–63. doi:10.1038/jid.2009.401. PMID 20054339.

[135]   Roschek B Jr, Fink RC, McMichael M, Alberte RS. Nettle extract (Urtica dioica) affects key receptors and enzymes associated with allergic rhinitis. Phytother Res. 2009 Jul;23(7):920-6. doi: 10.1002/ptr.2763.

[136]   C. Randall et al. Nettle sting of Urtica dioica for joint pain — an exploratory study of this complementary therapy. Complementary Therapies in Medicine, Volume 7, Issue 3, September 1999, Pages 126–131.

[137]   Johri RK and Zutshi U. Effect of quercetin and Albizzia saponins on rat mast cell. Indian J Physiol Pharmacol. 29(1). 43-6. 1985.

[138]   Tripathi RM and Das PK. Studies on Anti-Asthmatic and Anti-Anaphylactic Activity of Albizzia lebbeck. Ind. J. Pharmac. 9 (3). 189-1 94. 1977.

[139]   Agarwal et al. Herbal composition having antiallergic properties and a process for the preparation therof. United States Patent. 2004.

[140]   Michael, Paul. Herbal Medicines to Reduce the Excitatory Effect of Histamine and Treat Allergic Conditions. July 2009. Positive Health;Jul2009, Issue 160, p5

[141]   Loon VIM. The golden root: clinical applications of Scutellaria baicalensis GEORGI flavonoids as modulators of the inflammatory response. Alternative Medicine Review. 2(6). 472-80. 1997.

[142]   Hsieh et al. Baicalein inhibits IL-1β- and TNF-α-induced inflammatory cytokine production from human mast cells via regulation of the NF-κB pathway. Clin Mol Allergy. 5: 5. 2007.

[143]   Nishibe, Sansei & Murai, Michiko. Bioactive Components of Plantago Herb. The Japan Food Chemical Research Foundation.Faculty of Pharmaceutical Sciences, Health Sciences University of Hokkaido, Japan. Retrieved January 2014.

[144]   Samuelsen, Anne Berit. The traditional uses, chemical constituents and biological activities of Plantago major L. A review. Journal of Ethnopharmacology, Volume 71, Issues 1–2, July 2000, Pages 1–21.

[145]   Yoshikawa M, Shimada H, Shimoda H, Murakami N, Yamahara J, Matsuda H. Bioactive constituents of Chinese natural medicines. II. Rhodiolae radix. (1). Chemical structures and antiallergic activity of rhodiocyanosides A and B from the underground part of Rhodiola quadrifida (Pall.) Fisch. et Mey. (Crassulaceae). Chem Pharm Bull (Tokyo). 1996 Nov;44(11):2086-91.

[146]   Yoshikawa M, Shimada H, Shimoda H, Matsuda H, Yama-hara J, Murakami N. Rhodiocyanosides A and B, new antiallergic cyanoglycosides from Chinese natural medicine "si lie hong jing tian", the underground part of Rhodiola quadrifida (Pall.) Fisch. et Mey. Chem Pharm Bull (Tokyo). 1995 Jul;43(7):1245-7.

[147]   Pooja et al. Anti-inflammatory effect of Rhodiola rosea- 'a second-generation adaptogen'. Phytother Res. 2009 Aug; 23 (8):1099-102. doi: 10.1002/ptr.2749.

[148]   Lee, Yeonju et al., Anti-Inflammatory and Neuropro-tective Effects of Constituents Isolated from Rhodiola rosea. Evidence-Based Complementary and Alternative Medicine. Volume 2013 (2013), Article ID 514049, 9 pages. http://dx.doi.org/10.^{1155}/$_{2013}$/514049

[149]   Noli C, Carta G, Cordeddu L, Melis MP, Murru E, Banni S. Conjugated linoleic acid and blackcurrant seed oil in the treat-ment of canine atopic dermatitis: a preliminary report. Vet J. 2007 Mar;173(2):413-21. Epub 2006 Feb 21.

[150]   Garbacki et al. Proanthocyanidins, from Ribes nigrum leaves, reduce endothelial adhesion molecules ICAM-1 and VCAM-1. J Inflamm. (Lond). 2: 9. 2005.

[151]   Nirmala, P. 1and Selvaraj, T. Anti-inflammatory and anti-bacterial activities of Glycyrrhiza glabra. L. Journal of Agri-cultural Technology 2011,Vol. 7(3):815-823 815

[152]   Tamura, Yoshifumi & Nishibe, Sansei. Changes in the Con-centrations of Bioactive Compounds in Plantain Leaves. J Agric Food Chem. 2002 Apr 24;50(9):2514-8.

[153]   Marcucci MC. Propolis: Chemical composition, biological properties and therapeutic activity. Apidologie. 1995;26:83–99.

[154] Simone-Finstrom, Michael; Spivak, Marla (May-June 2010). "Propolis and bee health: The natural history and significance of resin use by honey bees". Apidologie 41 (3): 295–311. doi:10.1051/apido/2010016.

[155] Walker, Matt (23 July 2009). "Honeybees sterilise their hives". BBC News. Retrieved 2009-07-24.

[156] Author unknown. Saiboku-to Natural Standard, www.naturalstandard.com 2013. Retrieved january 2014

[157] Toda S, Kimura M, Ohnishi M, Nakashima K. Effects of the chinese herbal medicine "Saiboku-to" on histamine release from and the degranulation of mouse peritoneal mast cells induced by compound ^{48}/$_{80}$. J Ethnopharmacol. 1988 Dec;24(2-3):303-9.

[158] Author unknown. Asthma Care and Breathing Exercises Guide for Smartphones and Mobile Devices. ISBN: 9781605011158. MobileReference, 2010.

[159] Author unknown. Cortisone shots. MayoClinic.com. 2010-11-16. Retrieved July 31, 2013.

[160] Author unknown. Prednisone and other corticosteroids: Balance the risks and benefits. MayoClinic.com. 2010-06-05. Retrieved 2011-09-03.

[161] Jung, Min Kyung; Hur, Dae Young; Song, Seok Bean; Park, Yoorim; Kim, Tae Sung; Bang, Sa Ik; Kim, Seonghan; Song, Hyun Keun; Park, Hyunjeong; Cho, Dae Ho (2010). "Tannic Acid and Quercetin Display a Therapeutic Effect in Atopic Dermatitis via Suppression of Angiogenesis and TARC Expression in Nc/Nga Mice". Journal of Investigative Dermatology 130 (5): 1459–63. doi:10.1038/jid.2009.401. PMID 20054339.

[162] Zhang M, Swarts SG, Yin L, Liu C, Tian Y, Cao Y, Swarts M, Yang S, Zhang SB, Zhang K, Ju S, Olek DJ Jr, Schwartz L, Keng PC, Howell R, Zhang L, Okunieff P. Antioxidant properties of quercetin. Adv Exp Med Biol. 2011;701:283-9. doi: 10.$^{1007}/_{978}$-1-4419-7756-4_38.

[163] Zuyi Weng, Bodi Zhang et al, Quercetin Is More Effective than Cromolyn in Blocking Human Mast Cell Cytokine Release and Inhibits Contact Dermatitis and Photosensitivity in Humans. PLOS One. Published: March 28, 2012. DOI: 10.1371/journal.pone.0033805

[164] Davis JM, Murphy EA, Carmichael MD, Davis B (April 2009). "Quercetin increases brain and muscle mitochondrial biogenesis and exercise tolerance". Am. J. Physiol. Regul. Integr. Comp. Physiol. 296 (4): R1071–7. doi:10.1152/ajpregu.90925.2008. PMID 19211721.

[165] Balabolkin II, Gordeeva GF, Fuseva ED, Dzhunelov AB, Kalugina OL, Khamidova MM (1992). "Primenenie vitaminov pri allergicheskikh zabolevaniiakh u deteĭ" [Use of vitamins in allergic illnesses in children]. Vopr. Med. Khim. (in Russian) 38 (5): 36–40. PMID 1492394.

[166] Shaik YB, Castellani ML, Perrella A, Conti F, Salini V, Tete S, Madhappan B, Vecchiet J, De Lutiis MA, Caraffa A, Cerulli G. Role of quercetin (a natural herbal compound) in allergy and inflammation. J Biol Regul Homeost Agents. 2006 Jul-Dec;20(3-4):47-52.

[167] Author unknown. Quercetin. University of Maryland Medical Center, www.umm.edu/health/medical/altmed/supplement/quercetin Retrieved January 2014

[168]   Orsi, R. O.; Sforcin J. M., Rall V. L. M., Funari S. R. C., Barbosa L., Fernandes JR A. (2005). "Susceptibility profile of Salmonella against the antibacterial activity of propolis produced in two regions of Brazil". Journal of Venomous Animals and Toxins including Tropical Diseases 11 (2): 109–16. doi:10.1590/S1678-91992005000200003. Retrieved 2008-01-14.

[169]   Cafarchia C, De Laurentis N, Milillo MA, Losacco V, Puccini V (1999). "Antifungal activity of Apulia region propolis". Parassitologia 41 (4): 587–590. PMID 10870567.

[170]   Hoşnuter, M.; Gürel A., Babucçu O., Armutcu F., Kargi E., Işikdemir A. (March 2004). "The effect of CAPE on lipid peroxidation and nitric oxide levels in the plasma of rats following thermal injury". Burns 30 (2): 121–5. doi:10.1016/j.burns.2003.09.022. PMID 15019118.

[171]   Ocakci, A.; Kanter M., Cabuk M., Buyukbas S. (October 2006). "Role of caffeic acid phenethyl ester, an active component of propolis, against NAOH-induced esophageal burns in rats". Int J Pediatr Otorhinolaryngol. 70 (10): 1731–9. doi:10.1016/j.ijporl.2006.05.018. PMID 16828884.

[172]   Brätter, C.; Tregel M., Liebenthal C., Volk H. D. (October 1999). "Prophylactic effectiveness of propolis for immunostimulation: a clinical pilot study". Forsch Komplementarmed. 6 (5): 256–60. PMID 10575279.

[173]   Ansorge, S.; Reinhold D., Lendeckel U. (July–August 2003). "Propolis and some of its constituents down-regulate DNA synthesis and inflammatory cytokine production but induce TGF-beta1 production of human immune cells". Z Naturforsch [C]. 58 (7–8): 580–9. PMID 12939048.

[174]   Shinmei Y, Yano H, Kagawa Y, Izawa K, Akagi M, Inoue T, Kamei C. Effect of Brazilian propolis on sneezing and nasal rubbing in experimental allergic rhinitis of mice. Immunopharmacol Immunotoxicol. 2009;31(4):688-93. doi: 10.$^{3109}/_{08923970903078443}$.

[175]   Nakamura R, Nakamura R, Watanabe K, Oka K, Ohta S, Mishima S, Teshima R. Effects of propolis from different areas on mast cell degranulation and identification of the effective components in propolis. Int Immunopharmacol. 2010 Sep;10(9):1107-12. doi: 10.1016/j.intimp.2010.06.013. Epub 2010 Jun 29.

[176]   Lopes-Rocha R, Pereira EM, Marinho SA, de Miranda JL, Lima NL, Verli FD. Effect of propolis on mast cells in wound healing. Barroso PR, Inflammopharmacology. 2012 Oct;20(5):289-94. doi: 10.1007/s10787-011-0105-5. Epub 2011 Dec 17.

[177]   Botushanov, P. I.; Grigorov G. I., Aleksandrov G. A. (2001). "A clinical study of a silicate toothpaste with extract from propolis". Folia Med (Plovdiv) 43 (1–2): 28–30. PMID 15354462.

[178]   Koo, H.; Cury J. A., Rosalen P. L., Ambrosano G. M., Ikegaki M., Park Y. K. (November–December 2002). "Effect of a mouthrinse containing selected propolis on 3-day dental plaque accumulation and polysaccharide formation". Caries Research 36 (6): 445–8. doi:10.^{1159}/000066535. PMID 12459618.

[179]   Dodwad, Vidya and Kukreja, Bhavna Jha. Propolis mouthwash: A new beginning. J Indian Soc Periodontal. 2011 Apr-Jun; 15(2): 121-125.

[180]   Kumazawa, Shigenori; Hamasaka, Tomoko & Nakayama, Tsutomu. Antioxidant activity of propolis of various geographic origins. Food Chemistry. Volume 84, Issue 3, February 2004, Pages 329–339.

[181]   Frozza CO, Garcia CS, Gambato G, de Souza MD, Salvador M, Moura S, Padilha FF, Seixas FK, Collares T, Borsuk S, Dellagostin OA, Henriques JA, Roesch-Ely M. Chemical characterization, antioxidant and cytotoxic activities of Brazilian red propolis. Food Chem Toxicol. 2013 Feb;52:137-42. doi: 10.1016/j.fct.2012.11.013. Epub 2012 Nov 19.

[182]   Russo A, Longo R, Vanella A. Antioxidant activity of propolis: role of caffeic acid phenethyl ester and galangin. Fitoterapia. 2002 Nov;73 Suppl 1:S21-9.

[183]   Vickerstaff Health Services, 'About Dr. Joneja' www.allergynutrition.com. Retrieved January 2014

[184]   www.allergyuk.org. Retrieved January 2014

[185]   Swiss Allergy Centre www.aha.ch Retrieved January 2011

[186]   Miller MJ, Zhang XJ, Gu X, Tenore E, Clark DA. Exaggerated intestinal histamine release by casein and casein hydrolysate but not whey hydrolysate. Scand J Gastroenterol. 1991 Apr;26(4):379-84.

[187]   'Sago'. www.rbgsyd.nsw.gov.au/plant_info/talking_plants/ Retrieved January 2014

[188]   Hahn, S.K. An overview of traditional processing and utilization of cassava in Africa. FAO Corporate Document Repository. Proceedings of the IITA/ILCA/University of Ibadan Workshop on the Potential Utilization of Cassava as Livestock Feed in Africa, 14-18 November 1988.

[189]   Wikipedia. Cassava. Retrieved January 2014

[190]   Gupta Sonika, Gupta et al., Comparative Studies on Anti-Inflammatory Activity of Coriandrum Sativum, Datura Stramonium and Azadirachta Indica. ASIAN J. EXP. BIOL. SCI., VOL 1 (1) 2010: 151-154

[191]   Boskabady, M.H. et al., Relaxant effect of Cuminum cyminum on guinea pig tracheal chains and its possible mechanism(s). Indian Journal of Pharmacology. DOI: $10.^{4103}/_{0253}$-7613.15111

[192]   Wöhrl S, Hemmer W, Focke M, Rappersberger K, Jarisch R. Histamine intolerance-like symptoms in healthy volunteers after oral provocation with liquid histamine. Allergy Asthma Proc. 2004 Sep-Oct;25(5):305-11.

[193]   Grains with the Highest Protein to Carbohydrate Ratio. www.healthaliciousness.com   Sourced from USDA National Nutrient Database for Standard Reference, Release 20.

[194]   Gorski, Barb; Sustainable Agriculture Research and Education; Pastured Poultry Products. 1999

[195]   H1 antagonist—Wikipedia, the free encyclopedia. Retrieved January 2014

[196]   H2 antagonist—Wikipedia, the free encyclopedia. Retrieved January 2014

[197]   H3 antagonist—Wikipedia, the free encyclopedia. Retrieved January 2014

[198]   H4 antagonist—Wikipedia, the free encyclopedia. Retrieved January 2014

[199]   Food Challenge The Free Dictionary. Retrieved January 2014

[200]   Double Blind. The Free Dictionary. Retrieved January 2014.

[201]   Complementary Compounding Services. http://www.custommedicine.com.au. Retrieved January 2014

[202]   Akiyama H, Sato Y, Watanabe T, Nagaoka MH, Yoshioka Y, Shoji T, Kanda T, Yamada K, Totsuka M, Teshima R, Sawada J, Goda Y, Maitani T. Dietary unripe apple polyphenol inhibits the development of food allergies in murine models. FEBS Lett. 2005 Aug 15;579(20):4485-91.

[203]   Douglas Harper. Etymology Online. www.etymonline.com Retrieved January 2014.

[204]   Hedrick. U. P. Sturtevant's Edible Plants of the World.

[205]   Johnson. C. P. The Useful Plants of Great Britain.

[206] Harrington. H. D. Edible Native Plants of the Rocky Mountains.

[207] Saunders. C. F. Edible and Useful Wild Plants of the United States and Canada.

[208] Coon. N. The Dictionary of Useful Plants.

[209] Facciola. S. Cornucopia - A Source Book of Edible Plants.

[210] Weiner. M. A. Earth Medicine, Earth Food.

[211] Safe Homemade Flavored and Infused Oils. Food Safety: The University of Maine Cooperative Extension Publications. 2011.

[212] Nagao,Koji & Yanagita, Teruyoshi. Medium-chain fatty acids: Functional lipids for the prevention and treatment of the metabolic syndrome. Pharmacological Research Volume 61, Issue 3, March 2010, Pages 208–212

[213] Assunção, Monica L. et al., Effects of Dietary Coconut Oil on the Biochemical and Anthropometric Profiles of Women Presenting Abdominal Obesity. Lipids July 2009, Volume 44, Issue 7, pp 593-601

[214] Trinidad P. Trinidad et al., Glycaemic index of different coconut (Cocos nucifera)-flour products in normal and diabetic subjects. British Journal of Nutrition (2003), 90 , 551–556 DOI: 10.1079/BJN2003944

[215] Sagar Naskar et al., Evaluation of antihyperglycemic activity of Cocos nucifera Linn. on streptozotocin induced type 2 diabetic rats. Journal of Ethnopharmacology Volume 138, Issue 3, 8 December 2011, Pages 769–773

[216] Niebuhr. A. D. Herbs of Greece.

[217] Soda bread. Wikipedia, retrieved January 2014

[218] Ciabatta. Wikipedia. Retrieved January 2014

[219]   H. M. Kim and S. H. Cho, "Lavender oil inhibits immedi-ate-type allergic reaction in mice and rats," Journal of Pharmacy and Pharmacology, vol. 51, no. 2, pp. 221–226, 1999.

[220]   Sainty, Lane & Carroll, Lucy. Scombroid poisoning, linked to Noelene and Yvana Bischoff's deaths, rare. Sydney Morning Herald, February 5, 2014

[221]   Petersen LJ, Hansen U, Kristensen JK, Nielsen H, Skov PS, Nielsen HJ. Studies on mast cells and histamine release in psoriasis: the effect of ranitidine. Acta Derm Venereol. 1998 May;78(3):190-3.

Index

B

C

SYMPTOMS

About the Author

James L. Gibb is an educator, writer and health researcher with a particular focus on food-related diseases. A university graduate with a diploma of education, Gibb became interested in the relationship between nutrition and health when a family member was diagnosed with a chronic disease. He spent many years investigating natural alternatives to the powerful drugs prescribed for this condition, whose side effects can be damaging and debilitating. Over time he accumulated a wealth of information, which culminated in the writing of this book.

'Medical science has made enormous leaps in the 21st century,' writes Gibb, 'and without it, we would all be worse off. Dedicated medical researchers and doctors have improved our quality of life far beyond the standards available to preceding generations. That said, it is sometimes the afflicted themselves, or those closest to them, who are motivated to perservere just that little bit more keenly in pursuit of answers. Often, people with a personal investment in a health problem will stop at nothing to find a solution, seeking far and wide, never giving up.

' One example is the relentless quest of Augusto and Michaela Odone to find a treatment for their son Lorenzo's adrenoleukodystrophy, in the face of scepticism from health professionals. Their experience was later dramatized in the movie "Lorenzo's Oil". Another is provided by Elaine Gottschall, whose daughter was diagnosed with severe ulcerative colitis. Medications failed to improve the child's condition, and most doctors dismissed the idea that diet could be in any way associated with this digestive disease. It was a maverick doctor who thought 'outside the box' who finally led Ms Gottschall to a treatment for her daughter. When he died, to preserve his knowledge she wrote a book called 'Breaking the Vicious Cycle', which has been translated into several languages, and is published worldwide.'

'My own experience with a suffering child motivated me to search for answers even in the most unlikely places, which conventional medicine may overlook. Accepted medical opinion is far from infallible, as has been demonstrated from time to time, notably when Dr Barry Marshall swallowed Helicobacter pylori (H. pylori) bacteria to test the theory that they were a cause of peptic ulcer and gastric cancer. The H. pylori theory was ridiculed by scientists and doctors of the establishment, who did not believe any bacteria could live in the acidic environment of the stomach. Marshall has been quoted as saying in 1998 that "(e)veryone was against me, but I knew I was right."

'Sometimes it takes an outsider, unblinkered by conventional training, to perceive a truth. (After all, it was a humble clerk in the Swiss Patents Office who became the father of modern physics.)

'When the Strictly Low Histamine Diet had an almost miraculous effect on my own, seemingly unrelated symptoms I, too felt driven to share this knowledge with others.'

James L Gibb, 2014

Other best-sellers from Leaves of Gold Press

Beauty
The Ultimate Cosmetic Makeover Guide

By Elizabeth M Reed

People have been enhancing their looks with potions, plucking, dyes, paints, tattoos, corsets, wigs etc. since the dawn of the human race. In the 21st century, more sophisticated cosmetic techniques have become enormously popular, world-wide.

There is a vast and bewildering array of possibilities offered by an ever-burgeoning number of clinics and salons. Finding the perfect cosmetic treatment can be confusing. What treatments are available? Which of them best suits your needs?

The two books in the 'Beauty' series make the job of finding the appropriate cosmetic treatments quick and easy, for both men and women. We compare and describe dozens of beauty makeover techniques, from the most frugal and non-surgical to the most high-tech and dramatic.

Beauty: The Ultimate Cosmetic Makeover Guide
Book 1: Face and Skin

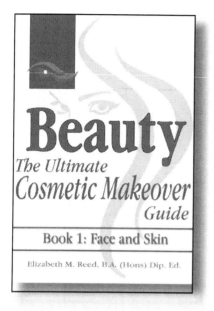

Volume 1 of the 'Beauty' series discusses cosmetic enhancements for the face and skin, including ways to boost collagen, diminish wrinkles, improve skin tone and color, tighten skin and rejuvenate the face.

Beauty: The Ultimate Cosmetic Makeover Guide
Book 2: Body, Teeth and Hair

Volume 2 of the 'Beauty' series looks at the numerous surgical and non-surgical techniques available for 'body sculpting,' such as fat transfer, liposuction, acoustic wave, fat freezing and laser therapies.

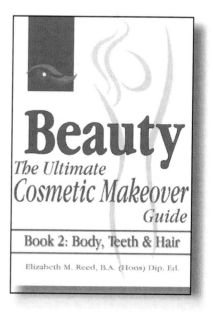

The Kitten Who Wants to Fall Asleep:
A Story To Help Children Go To Sleep

The #1 New Release in the category "Sleep Disorders".

Children sometimes find it hard to get to sleep.

What if you could read them a bedtime story incorporating powerful psychological methods to help them fall asleep quickly, easily and without drugs?

Psychological sleep induction techniques include:
- putting aside your thoughts until the following day
- breathing deeply
- slowing down
- visualizing a safe and peaceful place
- imagining a descent with the sensation of sinking
- progressive muscle relaxation
- using sleep-triggering words
- employing the 'infectiousness' of yawning.

Such methods are well-known and can be found in libraries or by searching for 'psychological sleep techniques' on the Internet.

This book also uses the hypnotic power of rhyme and rhythm. Songs and lullabies have traditionally been used to lull children to sleep. 'Hypnotic' poetry works in much the same way.

The poems in this book are in the relaxing, calming rhythm called 3/4 time, better known as 'waltz time'. All parents know that gentle, rocking rhythms can soothe a child.

The rhyming is as important as the rhythm. Children love poems that rhyme. For them, rhyming words make poetry fun and memorable.

Just as children respond to soothing rhythms and imagery, so they can fall asleep while listening to the tale of Misti the Kitty.

The Kitten Who Wants To Fall Asleep

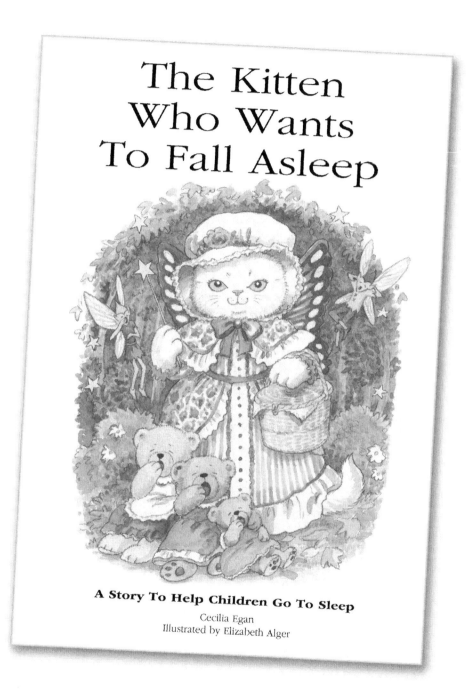

A Story To Help Children Go To Sleep

Cecilia Egan

Illustrated by Elizabeth Alger

www.leavesofgoldpress.com

NOTES

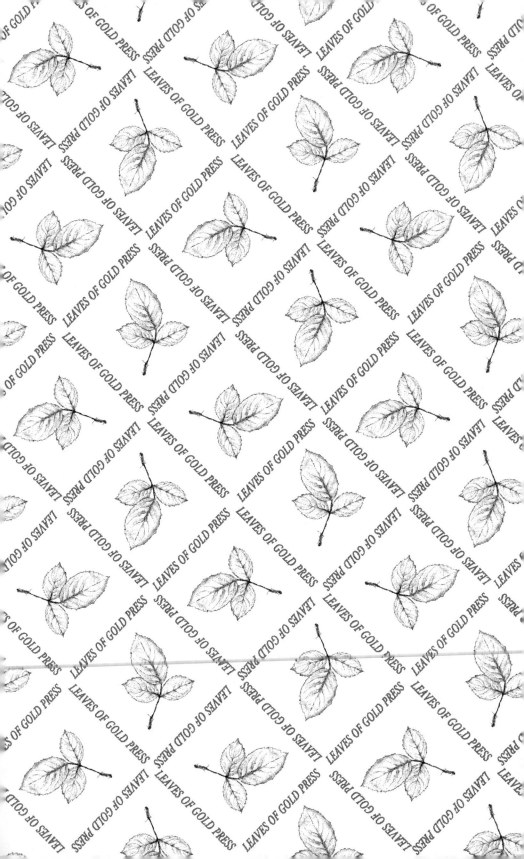

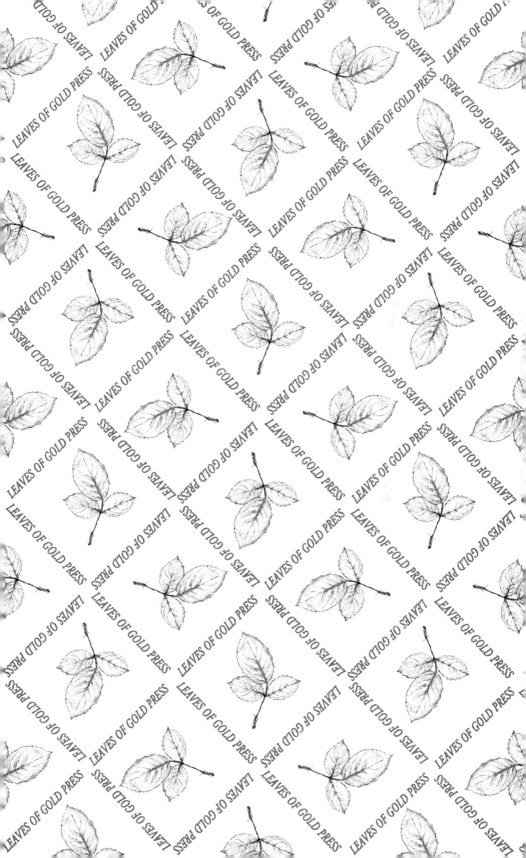

73758412R00206

Made in the USA
Lexington, KY
11 December 2017